FOREST BATHING

Also by Dr. Cyndi Gilbert, N.D.

The Essential Guide to Women's Herbal Medicine

FOREST BATHING

． ． ． ．

DISCOVERING HEALTH AND HAPPINESS THROUGH THE JAPANESE PRACTICE OF SHINRIN YOKU

{ A Start Here Guide }

DR. CYNDI GILBERT, N.D.

ST. MARTIN'S
ESSENTIALS
New York

FOREST BATHING. Copyright © 2019 by Cyndi Gilbert. All rights reserved. Printed in the United States of America. For information, address St. Martin's Press, 175 Fifth Avenue, New York, N.Y. 10010.

www.stmartins.com

The Library of Congress Cataloging-in-Publication Data is available on request.

ISBN 978-1-250-21448-5 (trade paperback)
ISBN 978-1-250-21449-2 (ebook)

Our books may be purchased in bulk for promotional, educational, or business use. Please contact your local bookseller or the Macmillan Corporate and Premium Sales Department at 1-800-221-7945, extension 5442, or by email at MacmillanSpecialMarkets@macmillan.com.

First Edition: May 2019

10 9 8 7 6 5 4 3 2 1

To the eastern white cedar and the redbud in my front yard,
who bring me shade, joy, and medicine in the heart of the city.

CONTENTS

4. FAQs

Appendix: Learn more

INTRODUCTION

Those who contemplate the beauty of the earth find reserves of strength that will endure as long as life lasts. . . . There is something infinitely healing in the repeated refrains of nature—the assurance that dawn comes after night, and spring after the winter.

—*Rachel Carson*

WHY YOU SHOULD TRY FOREST BATHING

Forest bathing isn't the kind of bath where you strip down and hop in a tub. You don't have to be naked to do it. At least, not necessarily naked. Forest bathing is about basking in nature, in greenery—and you can wear whatever you want. If you have ever sat under a tree or walked through the woods, you probably already know why you should try forest bathing. Each of us is intrinsically connected to the world around us, to nature. We are inspired by it, in awe of its vastness and wildness. Standing on a mountain ridge or looking out across the ocean underneath palm trees and mangroves, we are immediately struck by the way nature invites us to contemplate life, infinity, the universe, everything. This innate connection, or biophilia, often leads us to feel at home and relaxed in nature. Some people feel more grounded and steady, mirroring the roots of the trees. Other people sense clarity as they breathe deeper and more easily. Still others may feel protected and at ease from the smells of the trees, echoing the role these scents play in the lives of trees.

Over the past few years, forest bathing has surged in popularity in North America, alongside other quiet, minimalist activities such as *hygge* and the KonMari method of tidying up. Although the roots of forest bathing officially started in Japan, you don't have to travel far to feel the health benefits of standing among tree giants. You don't need any specialized gear or training to get started with forest bathing. In fact, some version of forest bathing has been an integral part of human lives in most places around the world since the dawn of time.

Forest bathing is a literal translation of *shinrin-yoku*, a term coined by the Japanese government in the 1980s to encourage urbanites to immerse themselves in nature to reduce stress and support overall health. The benefits of forest bathing go beyond the romanticism of Henry David Thoreau's *Walden* or the activism of John Muir. These days, there is hard science to support the claims of health benefits we've been hearing about for years.

Throughout human history, we've taken the benefits of being outside for granted. We spent most of our time outside, so there was no reason to think about why and how being in nature might actually be good for us. Or necessary. Now that we're inside more often than out, we're starting to realize that we need to be outside because we belong there. Spending too much time in the gray spaces of concrete buildings and sidewalks can have deleterious effects on our health. It can make us sadder, less active, more nearsighted, less focused, more stressed, and less capable of fighting off infections. On the other hand, spending more time in the green and blue spaces of the natural world can help to normalize blood pressure and blood sugar, build resilience to stress, increase vitamin D stores, encourage healthy aging, ameliorate mood, and enhance cognitive functions. It is these health-promoting and disease-preventing effects that have propelled forest bathing into popularity as a relaxation and stress management activity.

Imagine a therapy that is completely free, readily available, and virtually without side effects that can radically transform your health by improving your mental health, brain health, heart health, stress resiliency, immune system, and more. It exists, and it's called "nature exposure," or forest bathing. Interacting with nature is one of the most effective and easiest health hacks you can incorporate into your life. Learn why you should start forest bathing and how to do it. Better yet, take this book, sit under a tree, and start forest bathing right now.

HOW I GOT INTO FOREST BATHING

Since forest bathing is a phenomenon that started in Japan and has only recently made its way into the consciousness of the wellness movement in North America, people often ask me how I ended up writing a book about forest bathing. The short answer is, I'm a nemophilist. I am very fond of forests. I love the shade of the trees towering overhead, the mossy ground, the lichen growing on the sides of tree trunks, the plants in the undergrowth, the sound of the wind as it travels past the leaves, the smell of the forest after a rainfall. I am a haunter of the woods.

The longer answer is that although it's been less than ten years since I put a name to this practice, I've been forest bathing my whole life. I grew up in the suburbs of Ottawa, Canada, on a street lined with stately maple, pine, and willow trees. Our backyard was lined with thick cedar hedges, which were perfect places for secretly burrowing into during a game of hide-and-seek. We lived on the border of an area known as the Greenbelt, 49,400 acres (20,000 hectares) of protected green space, including farms, forests, and wetlands. Created in the 1950s to protect the rural land bordering the city from urban sprawl, it is the largest publicly owned greenbelt in the world. Growing up, I lived right next to it; it felt like an extension of my backyard.

A child in the forest

Some of my best memories of early childhood were in the forests near my home. Behind my elementary school, there was a forested area with a creek that ran through it. Technically, we weren't allowed to play there during recess, as it was outside the school boundaries, but I confess that my friends and I would venture there anyway, to play with sticks and watch spiders by the creekside away from the watchful eyes of teachers. In the winter, my family and I would go cross-country skiing on the Greenbelt trails. I was always in awe of the trees. Tall and majestic, the trees were home to adorable little chickadees in the winter that would chirp and eat seeds right out of my hand. It was magical.

I took trees and forests for granted. They were all around me. When I moved away from home to go to university, forests were still as omnipresent as they always were. My small, undergraduate university campus was on the outskirts of a medium-sized city, located along a river (Odoonabii-ziibi, or Otonabee, River). University campus buildings straddled the shores of the river, connected by a footbridge. Nestled in the woods, the university property included nature reserve areas and modern architecture designed to blend in with the natural environment. I pursued an undergraduate degree in cultural studies and took a deep dive into critical theory, looking at the ways in which the human body and nature are represented in our culture. Walking to classes felt like walking in a forest clearing beside the river, and I often found myself reading under a tree by the riverside, much as I had during elementary school.

When I got a job working for an environmental nongovernmental organization soon after graduation, it just made sense. I had spent my whole life surrounded by nature without thinking much about it, but I was also concerned about the environmental issues facing our world. I worked on projects that focused on the links between the environment, human health, and equity. I was a passionate champion for the communities and the people I worked with. They were people just like you and me who were affected by toxins in their neighborhoods, in their soil and air and water. I lobbied and fund-raised to protect and preserve forests and waterways, and I worked tirelessly on public education campaigns to increase everyday knowledge on the connections between the environment and human health. I was good at my job, but I knew that I was missing something. Deep in my gut I could sense that working in the environmental movement wasn't the right long-term career for me. I wanted to work more closely with nature in a positive way, but I wasn't quite sure how.

I had no clue what I was going to do, but I knew that I needed to take some space to figure it out. I got a job teaching English in southern China, a temporary move that I hoped would help me decide my next steps. The move to China did help me find clarity, in part because I moved to a large city without a tree canopy. I had to move away from forests in order to appreciate how much I needed them in my life.

Getting lost in the woods

Living in southern China was an amazing experience and also very challenging. It was on the other side of the world and drastically different from anywhere I'd ever lived or traveled before. I learned about living in a different culture; I learned a new language; and I learned a lot about myself. The city I lived in was a concrete-based urban center. There were no trees lining the residential streets, and only the most expensive gated condominium communities had any trees or gardens.

Southern China was also plagued by air pollution. The air was thick with black soot from the burning of coal and other combustibles. The floor of my apartment would get covered in a thin layer of black dust if I left the windows open during the day. I quickly learned that the slippers I thought everyone wore inside their houses for cultural reasons were also necessary for hygienic reasons. Within the first two months of living there, I got bronchitis. It was the first time I experienced firsthand the acute effects of air pollution. There was no respite from the smog and too few trees to help filter the air. I saw a traditional Chinese medicine doctor, who prescribed herbs to alleviate my cough and ease my breathing. The herbs worked tremendously well and I recovered quickly. I learned what foods to eat and which to avoid to help prevent getting sick again. Most important, the experience helped me to realize that I missed sitting underneath a tree beside the water. It was something I'd done all my life without thinking about it. It had never occurred to me how quickly my health would be affected when I didn't have easy access to a forest.

I did find a little oasis in that city, a small, private, treed park with a goldfish pond that I made an effort to visit for a couple of hours once every week or two. I also realized that I wanted to return to my roots as it were, to the healing power of nature that I instinctively understood as a small child lying in the grass under the maple tree in my front yard. I knew my next steps—to return to school to learn how to help others achieve better health through their connections with nature, from the use of herbal medicine and healing foods to the use of air, sun, water, and nature exposure. I searched for an educational program that could straddle arts and sciences and help me learn how to leverage our relationship to nature, to help others move on a path toward wellness. I searched for a university degree program that would guide me to a new career. A couple of months later I returned to North America, having been accepted into a naturopathic medicine program in Toronto, Canada.

I moved from a large urban city in China to Toronto, the largest city in Canada. In spite of urban developments, Toronto remains very green, with numerous ravines running through the city center. Even in the downtown core, the residential streets are often lined with large old trees planted more than one hundred years ago and punctuated by green space. The city's slogan, "A City Within a Park," is reflected in the presence of vast natural preserves at the city's eastern and western borders and the larger acreages that define entire neighborhoods such as High Park or

Riverdale Park, as well as the seemingly endless smaller parks that break up the urban landscape.

I got an apartment close to the subway, but also close to one of Toronto's smaller ravines. I reset my priorities so that I had a decent work-life balance while I was in medical school by making lifestyle changes that would ensure I had greater access to nature, even if I couldn't access a large forest. I didn't have a car, so I couldn't regularly travel to the conservation areas on the outskirts of the city. I made forest bathing happen, even if the forests I bathed in were rather small or were better defined as forested areas and small parks with a few trees. I walked or cycled to the subway through a park and went trail running through the ravine for exercise. Luckily for me, the naturopathic college was located on the edge of one of Toronto's largest rivers. Whenever I had the chance to take a break during school hours, I would go for a walk or a run along the riverside, soaking in the trees and the greenness. Forests and green space were once again part of my everyday.

Seeing the forest for the trees

I intuitively understood that being in forests was better for my health, but I was curious to find out more. Although the history of naturopathic medicine is full of doctors working out of clinics that doubled as health and wellness spas in the forests of Europe, I wasn't learning about the health benefits of spending time in nature in medical school. I attended classes in nutrition, herbal medicine, and hydrotherapy, but none of these courses taught me anything about the healing powers of just being in nature. Naturopathic medicine has its historical and linguistic roots in the word "nature," yet I spent most of my time in the classroom talking about foods and medicines that came from natural sources but rarely nature itself.

One of the guiding principles of naturopathic medicine is the *vis medicatrix naturae*, or the healing power of nature, but it was referenced in our classes only in history and philosophy. In those courses, I learned that medicine's history was full of doctors who considered nature to be the true healer. I read quotes attributed to Hippocrates and Paracelsus declaring that "nature itself is the best physician" and "the art of healing comes from nature." I contemplated the wisdom of the old Latin proverb *"Medicus curat, natura sanat,"* which translates to "The doctor cares, nature cures." I learned about doctors who eschewed the toxic and dangerous treatments prominent in their times, such as the use of arsenic compounds and bloodletting, in favor of treatments that focused on regular access to nature, hydrotherapy, healthy food, sunlight, and exercise. Their traditions, and their use of what many refer to as "nature cure," contributed to the history of naturopathic medicine as it was brought to North America and evolved into the profession it is today. Naturopathic doctors in the United States in the early 1900s often worked out of retreat centers or sanatoriums in the forest, so that their patients benefited from direct access to nature while receiving other forms of treatment.

Nature cure was great to learn about in theory, but I longed to learn more about the evidence supporting it. Instead, nature was treated in naturopathic medical school either as a historical artifact of the profession's early proponents or as simply the backdrop for other natural health treatments that were more tangible and easier to write on a prescription pad. So I looked into the research—I wanted to better understand how being in nature or not being in nature could impact people's health. I scoured research databases in my free time, reading study after study and concluding that lack of access to nature was associated with poorer health. On the flip side, I also found studies that supported better health and well-being from being in nature, even from looking at pictures of nature. Interest in concepts such as nature deficit disorder was just developing, and only a handful of people were talking about nature within medicine. I compiled hundreds of references and wrote academic articles and research papers that synthesized the research on nature and its relationship to different health outcomes. I spoke publicly at conferences for doctors, environmentalists, urban planners, and foresters. I regularly incorporated green prescriptions into my work with individual patients. My own experiences of improvements in my mental and physical health from being outside were validated by research and clinical studies. Most important, I practiced what I preached. I made sure that I spent lots of time forest bathing.

Forest bathing around the world

Anyone who knows me well knows that I plan most of my vacations around two things—forests and water. During summer family vacations, I love to paddle out in a canoe into the backcountry and camp for a few days in the Canadian wilderness, away from the hustle and bustle of the city. My favorite activities are just floating on my back in the water of a rock-bottom lake after a long canoe ride or swinging in the hammock that we've set up between two pine trees and looking up at the forest canopy. I am enamored of the way the light filters through the pine needles and the treetops appear to bend toward each other in an optical illusion. I love the creaking sound of the trees as they bend with the wind and the smell of the balsam fir and cedar trees. I could gently swing in the hammock for hours, if only my children didn't kick me out so they could have a turn too.

Most of my travel stories involve forest bathing of some kind or another. Often, I'll plan my vacations around trips to a new forest I've never visited or go out of my way to see a tree I've never met. A few years ago, I had a family wedding to attend in San Francisco. My children had spring break the week before the wedding, and since we were flying across the continent, we decided to make it a two-week road trip, driving from Los Angeles to San Francisco and back. Along the way, we stopped at Yosemite National Park to see groves of giant sequoias and coastal redwoods. After the wedding, we traveled south through Nevada to stand with the oldest living trees, the bristlecone pines. In both cases, we spent lots of time just standing among the trees, taking in the uniqueness of each forest and its beauty. I was so proud when my oldest, just eight at the time, was so inspired by our forest bathing experiences that he decided to write a short book on the incredible qualities of record-breaking trees.

Trees and forests are inseparable. Seeing a forest is to notice the trees that embody it. It means appreciating each individual tree for its own particular beauty. This year, while visiting the forests in Taiwan, I fell in love with a new-to-me conifer, the coffin tree (*Taiwania cryptomerioides*). Its name seems depressing, but looking at this tree revived my spirit. Historically, this tree's wood was used to make temples and coffins. Like many trees, the coffin tree reflects the deep connections between humans and trees. In some Indigenous communities in its range, a single tree would be chosen when a child was born and that tree would be carved to make that person's coffin when they passed away.

The coffin tree certainly stands out in a crowd. In the

aftermath of a summer downpour, the sweetness and clarity of the cypress-scented tree ushers in hope, joy, and calmness just as the rainbow after the rain. The bluish color of the needles reminds me of blue spruce, but it is the shape and fall of the branches that is most appealing and unique. The branches have a drooping or weeping quality but also form a dense, pyramidal shape. It gives the coffin tree the appearance of wearing a large-tiered, fringed flapper ball gown. I couldn't help smiling when I looked at this single tree.

And yet seeing a forest for the trees, as the saying goes, is to see the big picture and discern an overall pattern without getting tied up in the small details. When I'm forest bathing, it means I get a sense of the overall forest. Every forest is larger than the sum of its trees, and the experience of forest bathing is more than the individual types of trees. It's the sounds of the animals that live there, both on the ground and in the trees; it's the feel of the breeze against your face in rhythm with the swaying of the thinner trees. It's the smell of wet soil and rotting wood and the essential oils from conifers. It's everything added together, which creates an experience that is more than the sum of its parts. Sometimes forest bathing can even be transcendent.

Forest bathing can happen in unexpected places and ways. Sometimes you have to look around a corner to find something magical. Last year, I traveled with my family to Japan for vacation. After researching, writing, and speaking about forest bathing and the health benefits of getting outside for years, I finally had the opportunity to visit some of the forests just outside of Tokyo where forest bathing first began. My whole family was looking forward to exploring the bamboo groves just outside of Kyoto. We followed the hordes of tourists on the well-trodden path of the

Arashiyama Bamboo Grove. It was beautiful but extremely busy. The large number of people on the trail and the constant picture taking around us made it hard to truly appreciate the beauty of the bamboo forest. We were all a little disappointed.

We left the bamboo grove and went to visit a Shinto shrine, also in Kyoto, famous for its seemingly endless rows of red torii gates. At one of the shrines along the path, we stopped to use the bathrooms and found a side trail off the beaten track that we decided to explore. We turned a corner and suddenly found ourselves alone, on a path through a bamboo grove that rivaled the Arashiyama grove in beauty but without the swaths of people taking selfies. Rewarded with the forest bathing we were looking for, we had the entire path to ourselves. The four of us stood there, joyous in our discovery. We were automatically stunned into silence. The bamboo forest was unlike any we had ever been in. The visual beauty of the bamboo was striking. The culms, or bamboo stems, reached to the sky and were spaced evenly across the flat ground, with only sparse grasses in the spaces between them. The sound of the forest was even more incredible. Without the constant chatter of tourists and the clicking sounds of camera shutters, we could actually hear the creaking of the tall, skinny bamboo trunks and the hollow musicality of the trunks as they knocked together in the gentle breeze. The soundscape was a natural meditative backdrop. This sense of stillness, presence, and silence is universal to forest bathing no matter where in the world you are. Even my kids, usually skipping and laughing on a path in the woods, were spontaneously and suddenly silent and perfectly still. Finally, we were forest bathing again.

The place I feel most at home is in the coniferous forests of the Great Lakes region on the Canadian Shield. If you could see my true spirit, you would find it sitting on a granite rock over-looking the blue-green color of the limestone-bottomed lake as it reflects the forest green of a jack pine tree in its water. If you could hear it, it would echo the flutter of trembling aspen leaves, the lulling call of the loon, or the chickadee chirps that sound like "cheeseburger." If you could smell it, it would be the smell of cedar and spruce after the rain. If you could taste it, it would be the refreshment of wintergreen and the tartness of wild blueberry. If you want to find me, I'll be in the forest.

Green prescriptions

Forest bathing is my "outpatient department." As a naturopathic doctor, I often talk about forest bathing with my patients. Naturopathic medicine is holistic and looks at the big picture of someone's health. It takes into consideration the ways that health and illness are affected by everything from diet and exercise to mental-emotional factors and the environment. I ask almost all my patients about their exposure to nature, how often they go to a park or another natural environment. More often than not, my patients tell me that they spend little time outside. They lead busy lives, working and spending time with their partners, their children, or their aging parents. They travel by public transit or by car to their jobs. They prepare meals for their families, clean their houses, answer too many emails, shuttle their kids around the city for appointments or activities, and generally feel exhausted by the end of the day. They try to eat healthy and get enough exercise, usually at the gym, but they find themselves still struggling with losing weight or indigestion or anxiety or high blood pressure or depression or frequent colds and flus or insomnia or asthma. They are trying to do all the "right" things for their health, but they have a sense that something is missing.

When I ask about their relationship to nature, often they have that "aha" moment when they realize the missing piece of their health puzzle. Others respond with a nostalgic story about how much they loved a time or place in their life when they were around trees more often. Sometimes they just note that they wish they could find time to go to the park or go camping more often. Although most of my patients find it a challenge to incorporate forest bathing into their busy lives, they also know how important it can be for their health. Most people have their own stories about how nature exposure, or the lack of it, has impacted their health. Most of them intrinsically and intuitively understand that some connection isn't quite intact or has been lost.

How I incorporate green prescriptions varies greatly from patient to patient, depending on health concerns, lifestyle, mobility, and other factors. My urban office has a hidden garden filled with native medicinal plants and trees that frequently acts as an extension of my waiting room. In good weather, some patients choose to consult with me about their health concerns outside, sitting under the shade of the plum tree or next to the archway covered in raspberry and blackberry vines. When possible, we might conduct some or all of an appointment on a walk from my office to a local park, catching up on their health concerns or using the time for an individualized one-on-one forest bathing session. Even if we have to sit inside, the walls are mostly decorated with photographs of natural landscapes from around the world, filling the office with greens and blues. The waiting room is infused with essential oils of cedar, neroli, and pine.

Patients walk out of my office with clear guidelines and individualized plans for incorporating nature into their busy lives. These green prescriptions are a direct reflection of the science behind forest bathing and the unique way that I integrate forest bathing with other naturopathic health hacks. It isn't uncommon for me to write "Sit beside a tree" or "Go to the park" on my prescription pad. I can also be more specific about the particular variety of trees to seek out that corresponds to a particular patient's health concerns or that I have recommended be used for its herbal medicine qualities internally or topically. I might recommend that a patient use that time underneath a tree to listen to a guided meditation to help calm anxiety or improve concentration at work or school. For patients with fatigue, I might recommend dew walking first thing in the morning to help energize them for all that they want to accomplish in the day ahead. For those who also need more exercise, I might recommend they adjust their route to the subway to walk through a park or a street lined with big old trees. No matter what green prescription I might write down, my patients trust that I've based my recommendations on the clinical research and experiential knowledge confirming that forest bathing can have a positive impact on their health. As the anonymous quote frequently misattributed to French philosopher Voltaire (1694–1778) states, "Physic [medicine] is the art of amusing the patient while nature cures the disease."

{ 1 }

WHAT IS FOREST BATHING

ORIGINS

Forest bathing, the literal translation of the Japanese term 森林浴 *shinrin-yoku*, is described as the process of "making contact with and taking in the atmosphere of the forest." The term was coined in the early 1980s when the Forestry Agency of Japan proposed the promotion of forest bathing trips as part of a healthy lifestyle. Meetings were held to develop and nurture forest bathing as a relaxation and stress management activity. Forest bathing was promoted for its calm, quiet environment and clean, fresh air in contrast with the dense, loud urban conditions endured by many Japanese living in Tokyo and other cities.

Even though people in Japan and elsewhere around the world have been hanging out in forests since the dawn of time, the official naming and development of infrastructure around forest bathing is relatively new. Economic interests may have had a role in the development of forest bathing practice as we know it today. Forests and forestry have long been a part of the Japanese economy. Silviculture, or forestry, was a well-developed industry, growing stands of aromatic trees for both architectural and ceremonial uses. Leading up to the 1980s, there was interest within the forestry industry to support native Japanese tree stocks over imported wood products from neighboring Asian countries. Combined with academic research investigating the chemical compounds in conifer trees that give forests their characteristic smell, forest bathing made sense economically, culturally, and scientifically.

In 2004, the Japanese Ministry of Agriculture, Forestry, and Fisheries met with several academic groups and nonprofit agencies to begin to build up the research evidence on the health benefits of forest bathing. The concept of forest bathing brought together forestry and park departments with health and welfare departments, once separated as distinct and unrelated research and policy areas. This team, the Forest Therapy Study Group, conducted multiple research studies over the next three years, looking at everything from stress hormones and blood pressure to immune function and cognition. Out of that research, several academic institutes and nonprofit organizations were founded and became critical voices in advancing forest bathing practice.

The Society of Forest Medicine originated in 2007, born out of the Japanese Society for Hygiene, and is now housed with Nippon Medical School in Tokyo. Its mission is to advance forest bathing research and the therapeutic effects of forests on human health. It also works with businesses, governments, and universities to encourage the practice of forest bathing for health promotion.

Another organization, the Forest Therapy Society in Japan, also emerged from the research team in 2004. The Forest Therapy Society was tasked primarily with developing projects and public awareness to put forest bathing research into use. The society created Forest Therapy Bases to serve as centers for forest bathing practice and research and worked to raise public awareness of the health benefits of forest bathing. There are currently sixty-two Forest Therapy Bases in Japan, with plans to increase that number to one hundred bases. The Forest Therapy Society certifies and registers officially recognized Forest Therapy Bases and Therapy Roads. The organization also trains forest therapists or guides to lead people through a forest bathing experience. Their goal is to welcome and introduce as many people as possible to forest bathing. The majority of sites are barrier free and wheelchair accessible. Partnerships with local businesses support research and improve access. Corporations often subsidize forest bathing trips and may even include basic health checks.

Cultural and spiritual traditions also support the public promotion of *shinrin-yoku* and forest therapy. The traditions of gardening and meditation in Japan mirror the mindfulness part of the *shinrin-yoku* experience and may contribute to public acceptance and understanding of the practice. Japanese culture has long been characterized by a strong appreciation for nature and a harmonious attitude of connection to the natural world. Often depicted in modern times through the aesthetics of traditional Japanese gardens and a particular fondness for taking selfies in front of cherry blossoms, the cultural representations of nature connection can be equally found in the patterns on kimono fabrics or in the art of re-creating forest landscapes through the careful cultivation of miniaturized potted trees (*bonsai*) or the creation of tray landscapes (*bonkei*). Traditionally, nature themes have also been prevalent in Japanese architecture, art, cooking, and literature. Both Buddhism and Shintoism, the two most prominent religions in Japan, consider humans to be essentially identical to other parts of nature. Mountains, forests, plants, and animals are all embodied with spirits similar to those of humans. Although forest bathing was a relatively new practice, it was easily adopted likely because it was firmly embedded within the long-standing and widespread Japanese cultural identification with nature.

MOVING ABROAD / COMING TO AMERICA

While Japanese researchers were studying the health effects of *shinrin-yoku*, journalist and author Richard Louv was coming up with a new term of his own that would help set the stage for the introduction of forest bathing in North America. A columnist for *The San Diego Union-Tribune*, Louv documented a vanishing relationship with nature in his bestselling book *Last Child in the Woods: Saving Our Children from Nature-Deficit Disorder*. Louv argued that after tens of thousands of years of playing primarily outside in nature, children were increasingly living their lives indoors, and they were suffering because of it. He summarized and synthesized the research into the physical and mental health implications of staying inside.

The idea of nature deficit disorder hit a nerve. People like my patients started to think about how much free playtime they'd had outside compared with that of their own children and grandchildren. They thought about all the time they had spent outdoors themselves as children. They remembered feeling free to run around in the woods or on the open grassy areas. Like me, they had positive memories of playing outside, climbing trees, running with friends, picking up sticks, and walking far distances to school. They thought about their children and grandchildren and came to the realization that they were likely missing out on something without even knowing it. They became conscious of the fact that their children and grandchildren spent most of their time indoors, many of them in front of a screen. Their children couldn't identify and name a willow or a pine or even a maple tree. They were engaged mostly in structured, organized activities, mostly inside a building. In contrast, these adults, only one or two generations past, could fondly recall all the unstructured time they had spent wandering and getting dirty. They wondered about the effects of missing out on time spent in nature.

Others shared these concerns from professional perspectives. Urban and suburban planners had been talking about how to integrate trees into urban and suburban designs in new ways. The older, wealthier neighborhoods often still had a lot of streets lined with tall, mature trees, but the newer developments and less economically rich areas lacked the canopies of shade commonly found in other neighborhoods. City planners turned their attention to initiating and developing new forms of green spaces throughout cities, with active tree planting to replace aging canopies in the creation of greener, more livable communities for everyone. They also stressed the importance of nature-based solutions and renaturing cities to address nascent challenges of urban planning as more and more people moved into urban centers.

Environmentalists, conservationists, and naturalists had been raising alarm bells since Rachel Carson wrote *Silent Spring*, but there was an increased urgency in the 1990s and early 2000s. Concerns about the destruction of natural habitats and forests had existed for many decades, but public understanding and awareness and interest in these issues had greatly increased as the evidence of climate change accumulated. Scientific researchers had confirmed the cautions against the overharvesting of forests and the overuse of concrete in our cities. There was scientific consensus about the devastating impacts of climate change and air pollution.

Overall, the mainstream messaging had shifted. Organizations and cities started to invest millions of dollars into renaturalization efforts and planting trees. Artists and conservationists worked together to create new urban parks out of the ashes of old industry, such as the High Line in New York City. In my own city, an abandoned brick factory that sat unused along a ravine valley and the city highway that runs through it was converted into a green-designed hub and social enterprise for nature education, public art, and sustainable businesses. The renaturalized valley park now includes wetlands, wildflower meadows, and hiking trails as well as local markets, offices, an event space, and an outdoor skating rink. Every visit there is like stepping into another dimension where nature and the city shake hands and live in harmony. As with the High Line, where you can sit on a lounge chair under the tree canopy and gaze up at the Chelsea high-rises, the standard opposition of city and nature is disrupted by the space. It's hardly unusual to be standing next to the old brick chimney and watch a great blue heron swoop down into the wetlands area to go fishing. In the early spring, you can watch painted turtles slowly emerging from their hibernation, hidden in the mud on the pond floor still under a layer of ice, then turn around and watch the subway trains cross the valley on a bridge and hear the traffic on the highway.

Many other cities have initiated similar projects. Several cities in North America have renovated railway infrastructure into parkland, such as the 606 in Chicago, Illinois, or the BeltLine in Atlanta, Georgia. River restoration projects across the globe have been working to revitalize sections of urban rivers, such as the Los Angeles River in Los Angeles, the Milwaukee, Kinnickinnic, and Menomonee Rivers in Milwaukee, the Isar River in Munich, Germany, and the Cheonggyecheon in Seoul, South Korea. Overall, there is a movement afoot to develop livable cities that value nature as an integral part of social, economic, and environmental capital.

Organizations were founded to meet people's desire for nature reconnection and to drive policy changes to ensure the conservation of nature. Nonprofits such as the Children & Nature Network and the Child and Nature Alliance of Canada were created to focus on increasing children's access to nature. Other organizations sprouted up to focus on rewilding, renaturalizing, and teaching survival skills. The Rails-to-Trails Conservancy worked to transform unused rail tracks into multiuse trails. The Rewilding Institute and similar organizations centered on advancing wildlife conservation, while wilderness survival schools and forest therapy guided walks flourished. Older nongovernmental organizations such as the Sierra Club and the Nature Conservancy continued to work on conservation of the environment.

Reality TV shows such as *Survivor, Naked and Afraid*, Bear Grylls's *Man vs. Wild*, and Les Stroud's *Survivorman* inspired millions of people to rethink their relationships to natural spaces. Although many of those shows didn't shy away from highlighting the real dangers of outdoor existence and the accompanying fear, they also showed human perseverance and the ability to thrive under seemingly harsh conditions. Everything was coalescing toward a reconnection with nature through intentionally increasing nature exposure.

FOREST BATHING BY OTHER NAMES

You've probably already practiced forest bathing without even knowing it. Yes, forest bathing is catchy and it seems exotic because it has a Japanese name, but it isn't anything new to humankind. Even since the beginning of human time, we've had strong connections with nature. Obviously, at the very beginning, humans in hunting-gathering societies spent almost all of their time outside. Even with the introduction of agriculture, most of our time was spent outdoors, clearing areas for planting and working in the fields. We've come a long way since then, but it has been only a few generations since humans began spending the bulk of their time indoors. If you look around the world, you'll see that humans have developed different concepts similar to forest bathing to help frame the importance of getting outside for health.

Camping

Camping has a lot in common with forest bathing. In spite of how much work it can entail, camping is all about getting into nature and relaxing. Whether it's finding that perfect place for your tent or setting up a hammock between two trees or roasting marshmallows over a campfire or jumping into a lake or staring at the stars, the foundation of camping is nature appreciation. Ask campers why they camp, and the most common response you are likely to hear is that it's a great way to relax, escape the stress of daily life, and clear the mind while spending time with friends and family. People are camping for emotional well-being and health benefits.

It should come as no surprise that more people are camping more often. More than seventy-five million American households are camping at least once every year. Of those who camp, more people are camping overnight in national parks than ever before. Campers are camping more often and staying for multiple nights. Some people speculate that this renewed interest in camping has come about because staying in a tent is cheaper than other accommodation options. Others suggest that the increasing numbers of outdoor, multiday music festivals, mud runs, obstacle races, and other events have normalized camping for an entire generation, even if it isn't in the same style as traditional campgrounds.

Camping doesn't necessarily mean roughing it anymore, and neither does forest bathing. Although camping originally entailed going into the woods with little more than a tent and the ability to make a fire, camping has evolved to include comfort and even luxury. Nowadays, there are many different sleeping options in camping, from traditional tent camping to RV'ing to varieties of "glamping," a portmanteau of glamour and camping.

Camping and RV'ing today are an escape, an adventure, and a lifestyle. Unlike the basic practice of forest bathing, camping often includes other types of outdoor recreation. As much as campers spend time relaxing without exertion, they also spend a great deal of time moving their bodies. Today's campers tend to include more active forms of nature exposure, such as hiking, canoeing, fishing, rock climbing, and cycling. If you've ever gone camping, regardless of what activities you do once you're there, you've probably ended up forest bathing without even knowing it.

Spas and thermal waters

It may seem ridiculous, and even far removed from forest bathing as it has been practiced and researched in Japan, to talk about thermal spas in a book about forests. What does a spa have to do with forest bathing? you might ask. Everything. Taking forests out of their larger context serves only to segregate parts of nature. Forests are forests. Water is water. We draw an unnecessary and impossible line in the sand. We attempt to research the health benefits of forest bathing and compare it with water bathing. Which is better for your health—a green or blue environment? The answer is we'll never know. And we likely don't need to. Separating forests from their place within the natural world is the antithesis of forest bathing. Clearly, we've spent too much time in the forest noticing all of its minute details and have lost track of the bigger picture. We shouldn't forget that forests are made up of trees. Those trees depend on water. Trees in the mountains are fed by glacial springs. Trees in the valleys are fed by creeks, springs, rivers, and lakes. Trees depend on water sources. Even if you don't see them while forest bathing, they are always there, underneath the ground, providing nourishment through the forest floor.

I understood this intrinsic relationship between forests and water as a child, as I sat on the banks of a slow-moving river under the shade of a willow tree or on a granite rock next to a pine tree by a lake. I could feel the movement between wood and water as I sat, as an adult, in an outdoor hot pool in a spa in Chelsea,

Quebec, watching the weight of wet snow bear down and bend the cedar tree branches. I could feel the wholeness of nature and the interconnections among the elements—water, wood, air, earth, fire. Forests and the water that flows through them are inseparable, as much as we try to build fences around them in our minds.

Ever since the Neolithic period of history, humans have been immersing themselves in baths. Although the earliest humans likely indulged in thermal baths to stave off the bitter cold, later humans across the globe have incorporated bathing in hot and cold waters for hygienic, social, and spiritual reasons.

The earliest public baths on record were found in the Indus Valley and date back to 2500 BC in what is now Pakistan. Public baths were common in the ancient Greek, Roman, and Ottoman Empires, where cleanliness of the body and purification of the soul were the main reasons for bathing. Japanese *onsen*, Russian *banyas*, and Korean *jjimjilbangs* were similarly developed for benefits to health and spirituality. Many of these *thermae* or *balnae* (larger and smaller baths, respectively) were built into their natural surroundings so that the bath had a view of a forest, gardens, or mountain. Some had waters supplied by aqueduct, while others made use of the therapeutic thermal waters from natural hot springs.

In the late eighteenth century, doctors often prescribed hydrotherapy, the use of hot and cold water, as well as sunlight, fresh air, and gentle exercise for a variety of health conditions. Christoph Wilhelm Hufeland (1762–1836), royal physician to the king of Prussia, was influenced by many of the philosophers and poets in his time. Hufeland, and other doctors following him, espoused a natural, simple life, writing that a day spent in the country with friends and under a serene sky was better than any life-prolonging elixir in the world.

The movement to "return to nature" blossomed and thermal spas surged in popularity once again. Resorts were built around the baths that had been established earlier by the Romans in places such as Vichy (France), Baden-Baden (Germany), and the appropriately named Bath (England). Other spa towns developed in eastern European cities, where hydrotherapy was combined with therapeutic peat muds in places such as Karlovy Vary or Mariánské Lázně in the Czech Republic and Lake Hévíz in Hungary. People flocked to thermal spas to alleviate chronic pain and skin conditions, to promote circulation and even fertility. Not everyone who visited these spas was ill. As in earlier times, many people went to relax, socialize, and experience the therapeutic landscape. Although water was still at the center of treatments, wandering strolls through meadows and forests were also an integral part of the overall spa experience.

European spas, and increasingly spas in North America, are often a mix of forest bathing (either intentional or incidental) with other wellness, medicinal, and/or beauty treatments. Many of the older spa towns in the Alps or the Black Forest in Germany, the Czech Republic, and Hungary offer unique opportunities for variants on forest bathing, often in an upscale hotel resort but also with more modest accommodations. European campgrounds and other outdoor hospitality parks often mix camping in some form or another with wellness services such as saunas, pools, massage, hydrotherapy, and beauty treatments. Health tourism is on the rise as people look for different ways to escape city living and reconnect with the outdoors.

I'm no stranger to this type of tourism. While not every

thermal waters location is outside, many do make use of their surrounding landscape to amplify the experience. Last year, I visited the Tyrolean Alps in Austria for a child-free vacation of forest bathing, mountain hiking, adventure activities, and taking the waters. I confess, the thermal spa in town was the main attraction and driving force behind visiting this particular valley in the Alps. The spa is located on the valley floor, set below the towering snow-capped peaks. Several outdoor swimming pools allow you to soak, float, and drift in the thermal spring waters, with a 360-degree view of the conifers covering the slopes on every side. Forest bathing from the pool, or from a lush recliner with a glass of wine in hand, is the ultimate in luxury.

Likewise, North America is experiencing a renaissance of nature spas. Although the natural healing centers of the early 1900s, such as early naturopathic doctor Louisa Lust's Jungborn in New Jersey, have long since closed, new spas are popping up to meet the demand for outdoor, integrated nature spas. One of my favorite times to visit these spas is during the dark, cold days of winter in Quebec, just on the other side of the Ottawa River. During winter, it's easy for your mood to feel as frozen and your ambition as frigid as the temperature outside. The snow can feel as if it's dampened and paralyzed your heart. February can feel like forever, in spite of it being the shortest month of the year. Winter can also be cleansing and awakening and revitalizing. This refreshing side of winter is often characterized by the polar bear plunges, jumping into freezing-cold rivers and lakes, sometimes through rectangles cut out of the ice blanket layer on top. I prefer, however, a dip into a cold pool after a hot sauna, wearing a fluffy spa robe and flip-flops, walking on a stone path cut in the forest that separates the saunas, pools, and resting areas. As I rise out of the cold water, finding the outside air temperature almost tolerable by comparison, my body and mind feel alive and strong. Plus the conifer trees provide a deep green color that reminds me that spring will come once again.

Friluftsliv

Friluftsliv (pronounced free-loofts-liv) literally translates from the Norwegian as "free air life" or "open-air living." Although the term originates in Norway, it is a philosophy and cultural concept common to Scandinavian countries that prioritizes time spent unwinding outdoors. Popularized by Henrik Ibsen (1828–1906), the famous Norwegian poet and playwright, *friluftsliv* encourages time spent in nature for physical and spiritual well-being.

Friluftsliv is a way of life spent exploring and appreciating nature in an easy, uncomplicated fashion. Similar to forest bathing, *friluftsliv* prides itself on its simplicity. It doesn't require any equipment, and it doesn't hold to any preconceived notions of how to commune with nature. It's just about being outside. In this sense, *friluftsliv* is broader than forest bathing, since it can include going for a run at lunch, commuting to work on cross-country skis, sitting with friends and family in a sauna or mountain hut, and even ice fishing.

Connection to nature in Scandinavia comes naturally. Nordic countries are sparsely populated and nature is literally at your doorstep, or at least very close by. It's hard to ignore nature, since it's staring you in the face. *Friluftsliv* is a testament to Nordic peoples' relationship to the land. It is also closely tied to another Scandinavian concept, a law that codifies the rights of individuals to access the land, even private property, so long as they respect it.

Long before forest bathing was named as a practice, *frilufts-liv* was promoted by tourist and outdoor organizations in Sweden and Norway from the 1860s to the 1890s to help people cope with industrialization and urban development. The goal of *friluftsliv* was to foster good health through nature connections and the romanticism of old Scandinavian outdoor life traditions. The Scandinavian identity as a strong, nature-loving people was reinforced in the early 1900s through *friluftsliv* and outdoor activities.

Friluftsliv is so ingrained in Nordic culture that many employers and schools build time into their weeks to ensure that employees and students can spend time engaging in *friluftsliv*. Tax breaks are available in both Finland and Sweden for companies that subsidize their employees' activities. Government-tallied statistics in Sweden suggest that around one-third of all Swedes participate in an outdoor activity at least once a week.

Nowadays, *friluftsliv* may be somewhat more commercial, focused on activities and equipment over the philosophy of nature connection. No matter—being outside is good for you, no matter what you do or how you spend your time outside.

Related practices

Forest bathing isn't new and it isn't specific to Japan, or even to Asia. There are different practices and terms in many languages that highlight the relationship we have as humans with nature and the manner in which we interact with our environment in positive, health-promoting ways.

Think about going for a picnic. Picnicking is an activity that happens outdoors, sometimes while sitting on the ground, often underneath the shade of tree. To a certain extent, a picnic is forest bathing with food. It might be more social than forest bathing, as a get-together with family and friends. A picnic could also be more intimate, staged as a romantic outing. Taking an after-dinner walk is also a quiet, contemplative outdoor activity of the kind that forest bathing embodies. It is a time for digestion and a gentle stroll. Either way, both picnicking and after-dinner walks share some of their basic features with forest bathing—you are spending time outdoors, in nature, doing a relaxing activity.

Words in other languages can also provide clues to the important role of nature in specific cultures. *Dadirri*, a word that originates in the language of the Australian Aborigines, refers to the deep listening and still awareness that can arise from contemplating the quietude and beauty of nature. In Italian, the verb *meriggiare* means "to pass the hottest hours of the day outdoors in the shade." The German word *Waldbaden* literally means "to bathe in the forest" and is a newer word adopted to embrace the forest bathing movement and incorporate it within German culture. Other words refer to a specific observation about the natural world. *Petrichor* is a term first coined by Australian scientists in the 1960s that refers to the musty smell of rain as it falls on dry land. *Komorebi*, from the Japanese, means the light that dapples the forest floor as it is filtered through the trees' leaves.

Unique nature words can also describe a feeling rather than practice or an image. *Waldeinsamkeit* refers to the emotions that arise when you are in the forest by yourself for extended periods of time. Translated from the German, *Wald* means "woods" and *Einsamkeit* means "solitude." Even though the literal translation refers to solitude, *Waldeinsamkeit* doesn't equal loneliness. It generally refers to the enjoyment that arises after spending time in the forest, like the Ralph Waldo Emerson poem of the same name.

Waldeinsamkeit arises when you are strolling through the woods, appreciating the forest in all its beauty—the smell of the trees, the songs of birds, the gentle breeze, and the quiet, stress-free time. In other words, *Waldeinsamkeit* is the German word for the joy of forest bathing.

2

WHY YOU SHOULD DO IT

To be whole. To be complete. Wildness reminds us what it means to be human, what we are connected to rather than what we are separate from.

—*Terry Tempest Williams*

YOU BELONG OUTSIDE

We are part of nature—we belong in it. Don't get me wrong, I treasure the indoors and the ability to escape from the raccoons and skunks that occupy my backyard after dusk. I appreciate my access to air-conditioning during the sticky, sweaty thick of summer. I am eternally grateful for central heating when the thermometer drops to minus-22 degrees Fahrenheit (minus-30 degrees Celsius) and I can stay toasty warm inside. I also know that I need to spend time outside. Cabin fever is real, and I'm not interested in it.

Throughout human evolution, we've spent over 99 percent of our time in natural environments and under 1 percent of it in modern surroundings. Nowadays, over 70 percent of people in the United States live in urbanized areas, and we're spending less time in nature than ever before. Nature-based recreation in the United States has declined up to 35 percent in the past forty years. More than ever, a concerted effort is required to bring nature into our cities and to bring ourselves into nature.

We know that proximity to nature buffers stress and improves overall health in myriad ways. How green your neighborhood is corresponds directly to how happy you are to live in it. People living within 1.9 miles (3 kilometers) of dense green space are less likely to experience the negative impacts of stress and have fewer health complaints, even when faced with major losses, relationship problems, economic instability, and other stressful life events.

This difference in health outcomes is only amplified the closer or farther away from forests, parks, beaches, and lakes you live. People who live closest to green space are the least likely to get diagnosed with the most common chronic diseases. On the flip side, people living farther than 0.6 miles (one kilometer) away from green space are over 40 percent more likely to experience high stress. They score lowest on subjective measures of general health, vitality, mental health, and highest on measures of body pain. At the far end of the scale, people with less than 10 percent of green space within 0.6 miles (one kilometer) of their home are at 25 percent greater risk of depression and 30 percent greater risk of an anxiety disorder compared with people who had the largest percentage of green space within the same radius. The closer to green space you live, the healthier you are. The farther away, the greater your risk of illness and overall poor health. We need nature to live our best lives.

Using different words but similar values and concepts, most of the world's cultural traditions and religions express an affinity for nature. Forests and trees play an important role in Buddhism, where nature is regarded with a sense of reverence and is associated with joy, aesthetic beauty, spiritual freedom, and even enlightenment. Jean-Jacques Rousseau (1712–1778), the famous Swiss-born French philosopher, argued for a return to nature and wrote about "reverie," the blissful feeling of connection and loss of consciousness of the self when experiencing the wholeness of nature.

The drive to connect with nature has been described by biologist Edward O. Wilson as biophilia. Biophilia is the idea that an instinctive bond exists between humans and other living beings and systems. It is grounded in the knowledge that humans have a natural drive to commune with nature and that nature is critical in our development.

Intrinsically, most people know that they feel better in a natural setting, whether that's in the woods, on the beach, or on a mountaintop. That's why so many people gravitate to nature to relax and take a break from their daily routine.

NATURE DEFICIT DISORDER

Nature is not a place to visit. It is home.

—*Gary Snyder*

It's indisputable. We spend more time inside than ever before. Much of this change is for the better. We have better, though not universal, access to clean water in our homes, shelter from our environments, and information at our fingertips. More than 50 percent of us worldwide live in cities. Within the next several decades, 90 percent of North Americans and 70 percent of global residents are expected to live in urban centers. We can travel inside between buildings using underground walkways and subways. We can order food and supplies with the touch of a button and it will soon be on our doorstep. Modern conveniences are very convenient by design. They allow us freedom and efficiency and even health in many ways. Like all conveniences, however, there can be a cost. I'm not talking about a price tag, although some of our indoor life can be expensive. The health costs of indoor living are more elusive. It is something that is hard to measure and even harder to study.

Today's children, and many adults, are much less connected to nature than ever before. Why?

Much of it is by design. Many people live outside of the easy reach of nature. Looking out a window or opening their doors, they don't get to see trees. Many neighborhoods in dense large cities have more concrete and tall buildings and gray space than greens and blues. People living in low-income neighborhoods have even less access to green space. And people who are incarcerated are among the least exposed to nature.

Technology has also played a role. As children and adults spend more time on their screens, using technology for education and leisure, they spend less time outside. Excessive screen time is a risk factor for obesity, poor cognitive performance, anxiety, and depression. Sociocultural factors such as the way we design our cities or lack of transportation and safety concerns can also stop us from spending the amount of time in nature that we might want. Today, less than 10 percent of children regularly play in wild places.

Almost 50 percent of their parents, on the other hand, were part of a generation that spent time outdoors on a daily basis. Even when children do go outside, the area they are allowed to roam in has declined by almost 90 percent in a single generation. Nowadays, less than two-thirds of ten-year-olds have been to a shop or a park by themselves. In 1971, 80 percent of seven- and eight-year-olds traveled to school on their own. By 1990, that proportion was down to 9 percent.

The lack of time outdoors has had its negative effects. Vitamin D deficiency rates are high worldwide, and children aren't getting enough exercise. Almost 90 percent of Canadian children don't get ninety minutes of physical activity per day, the recommended amount to maintain a general fitness level. At the same time, lack of exposure has translated into a lack of knowledge about nature. A survey of children in the United Kingdom found that 50 percent couldn't tell the difference between a bee and a wasp, yet 90 percent of them could recognize a Dalek, a fictional extraterrestrial from the TV series *Doctor Who*. Because children spend less time outside, they have fewer regular, positive experiences in nature. We often fear what we don't know, and children are no different. Children who have exposure to uncomfortable or frightening views of nature, even if that exposure is on TV, may develop a fear of nature and avoid developing personal connections to the outdoors. The resulting eco- or biophobia can end up making the problem worse.

Children who play less outdoors may be less likely to try new things out in the open, less likely to test themselves and their limits. They might not try to walk across the fallen tree trunk that spans the creek or climb a tree or leap from one rock to another. Without taking chances and evaluating risk, they may be less likely to learn to cope with the challenges they'll face as adults in other areas of their life. They might not risk breaking a leg if they fall; instead, the risks they face may be a lack of confidence in themselves, the inability to make informed choices when there is a risk of harm, and a lack of resilience to stressful situations.

Richard Louv, studying the long-term effects of these changes in lifestyle, coined the term "nature deficit disorder" to describe the social, behavioral, and health costs of alienating ourselves from the natural world. Although scientists are just beginning to understand the health impacts of urban, mostly indoor living, one thing is clear: we need to put down our devices and get outside.

THE HEALING POWER OF NATURE

> I understood at a very early age that in nature I felt everything I should feel in church but never did. Walking in the woods, I felt in touch with the universe and with the spirit of the universe.
>
> —*Alice Walker*

Living in cities, we often feel disconnected from nature. Forest bathing helps us connect with the natural world as part of it, rather than being separate from it. Nature has a special healing power we can tap into. Step outside your door and you start to experience the healing power of nature. Walk into a forest and tap into a different kind of network.

Dating back to Hippocrates, the healing power of nature argues that there is an inherent and ordered tendency in nature toward balance and the restoration of health when things go awry.

It's reflected in the health of each individual being, from the smallest of bacteria to the largest of mammals. The healing power of nature is often defined as the ability of living things to heal themselves. It is reflected in the human capacity to heal wounds, to mount an immune response to a virus or a bacteria, to recover from traumatic events.

The healing power of nature can be found in the health of the ecosystem as a whole, too, a mirror of the healing power of nature found inside each person. This self-healing force exists within individual living things, as trees, too, regularly heal wounds caused by lightning or insects. The *vis medicatrix naturae* also exists between them, as evidenced by symbiotic relationships and fungal networks. It is within us, within other things, and between us. The healing power of nature can be seen as the glue that binds us together with nature, the rationale for our biophilia.

The healing power of nature can also be seen from another perspective. According to Sir John Arthur Thomson (1861–1933), a Scottish biologist and popular science writer, nature ministers to our minds. He held the belief that there exists deeply rooted and far-reaching interconnections between humans and nature that steady and enrich our lives. Without this alliance with nature, we cannot escape a feeling of loss and psychopathology. We can leave, head out on our own, build cities, and travel in underground tunnels, but we will always return to nature, like a home we return to after traveling abroad.

Health and healing, according to Thomson, is to be found in the mindful contact with nature. In his keynote address at the annual meeting of the British Medical Association in 1914, Thomson said, "We have put ourselves beyond a very potent *vis medicatrix* if we cease to be able to wonder at the grandeur of the star-strewn sky, the mystery of the mountains, the sea eternally new, the way of the eagle in the air, the meanest flower that blows, the look in a dog's eye."

Simply put, forest bathing is an opportunity to tap into the inherent healing power of nature—from encouraging a healthy microbiome to breathing oxygen-rich air. While Japanese researchers theorize that the essential oils, or phytoncides, in the forest air are responsible for many of the health benefits associated with forest bathing, phytoncides tell only part of the story. There is something more going on in our time spent outdoors—a sense of groundedness and interconnectedness that results from an attunement to the rhythm of nature and an awakening of the *vis medicatrix naturae* in each of us.

Nature is healing in part because it contains natural patterns that are harmonious and aesthetically soothing and similar to the patterns within us. The world is full of repetitive patterns, fractals that can be found in plants, animals, human anatomy, and even the shapes of galaxies. As one manifestation of the healing power of nature, fractals are found equally within us and within other aspects of nature. Fractals govern the formation of ice crystals and snowflakes, the arteries and veins in your body, and the structure of alveoli in your lungs. They are present in the branching of trees and rivers, as well as the buds of Romanesco cauliflower, pinecones, sunflower seed heads, and fiddleheads. Fractals are formed by infinitely complex mathematical patterns that look the same no matter their size or scale.

These patterns are beautiful, unique, and yet recognizable because they are found just about everywhere. We are innately fluent in the visual language of fractals because we are made up of similar patterns. We are hardwired to understand fractals and to respond to them in specific ways. Resonance with nature leads to physiological relaxation. When the world around us matches our insides, we feel safe and calm. Fractal patterns feel harmonious, pleasing, and comforting, like the rhythm of ocean waves, the flames in a campfire, or the spiral of a seashell. They have even been found to explain why people like certain works of art. Art and aesthetics researchers have shown that looking at fractals reduces the experience of stress, as measured through brain waves and electrical skin conductance. All this maps to the visual scanning patterns our eyes make when we look at forests and oceans and paintings by Jackson Pollock (well studied in the realm of fractal aesthetics). It turns out our eyes use search patterns that are themselves fractal in nature, patterns that mimic the search trajectories of nonhuman animals searching for food on land and in the air. Since fractals are so ubiquitous in nature, they may be one of the keys to understanding why forest bathing is so good for our health.

Then there's the oxygen, the fresher, less-polluted air. There's also vitamin D, which we get naturally only from exposure to the sun (unless we take supplements or fortified foods). Without adequate vitamin D, we increase our risk of developing many different diseases. Multiple sclerosis is found only at higher latitudes, where vitamin D is decreased. Vitamin D deficiency is so common in Canada that researchers and clinicians more or less assume that everyone is at least a little deficient and recommend supplementing daily.

Although we don't have all the words or tools to explain our connections, we understand instinctively that our health, from the biopsychosocial to the spiritual, is a reflection of the health of the earth. If we accept that human health and planetary health are one, then our moral and social obligations to restore a healthy and healing connection to our environment become imperative; they challenge us to rethink many of the ways in which we live, eat, work, and play. In so doing, we can foster and renew a mutually respectful relationship with nature. As nature heals us, we in turn can nurture and heal the planet; we can begin to truly appreciate the healing power of nature.

BUILD RESILIENCE

I go to nature to be soothed and healed, and to have my senses put in tune once more.

—*John Burroughs*

There is so much wisdom we can learn from trees. Trees are very adaptable, more often than not growing in less than ideal conditions and still managing to thrive. Trees can shift their leaves to absorb more or less sunlight depending on how shaded they are by their neighbors. They can grow shorter than usual, to the size of a bush, if they find themselves on a rocky, windy slope with little soil for their roots to hold on to. Trees can adapt and recover from pests or a particularly harsh winter, even if it takes them a few years. There are lessons here for humans to learn from if we are listening. Trees can teach us resilience and patience in the face of chronic stress or illness. As Rainer Maria Rilke wrote, "If we surrendered to earth's intelligence, we could rise up rooted, like trees."

Forest bathing has a positive impact on many markers of stress. It decreases blood pressure, anxiety, and stress hormones.

When we feel relaxed, we activate the parasympathetic nervous system, the opposite of our fight-or-flight response. We turn down the parts of our brains associated with executive functions such as organization, planning, and problem solving, while engaging the parts of our brains associated with pleasure and empathy. We can focus on digestion and the basics of metabolism.

When we're stressed, we activate the sympathetic part of our nervous system, commonly known as our fight-or-flight response. Our breathing becomes faster and more shallow. Our heart rate increases and our pupils dilate. We shunt blood away from our internal organs and into our muscles to help us get ready to run away from a bear or whatever dangerous thing is about to happen. We become more aware of our environment and focused so we can do whatever is necessary to stay safe. Behind the scenes, our body kick-starts this stress response by releasing three hormones—adrenaline, norepinephrine, and cortisol.

That system works just fine if you face only acutely stressful situations, such as when you're about to cross the street and then a car whips around the corner and you have to jump back onto the sidewalk to stay safe. It doesn't work as well when the stressful situation lasts for a long time and it seems like there's no way out. Low-grade, chronic stress, like the stress many people experience in their busy, working, urban lives, can wreak havoc on stress hormones. Depression, anxiety, and conditions such as post-traumatic stress disorder can have negative long-term health outcomes related to the physiological effects of stress on the body. Poor sleep, unhealthy diets, and even dysfunctional relationships can all affect the body's stress system and put the sympathetic nervous system into overdrive. It's one thing if your heart rate increases for a few minutes or even an hour and then goes back down to its lower, resting state; it's another thing if your heart rate and cortisol levels and breathing rate are raised for days or even weeks on end. Too much cortisol can suppress your immune system, increase blood sugar and blood pressure, contribute to obesity, and so much more.

Studies have looked at how forest bathing may help build resilience to stress and reduce the harmful effects of long-term exposure to stressful situations. Early research showed that exposure to nature provided relaxation. In those studies, participants said they felt better emotionally and that they recovered faster from stress.

Deep-dive research into how forest bathing works to relieve stress was important, especially since at least some of the impetus for the genesis of forest bathing was to alleviate the chronic stress of urban workers in Japan. Figuring out why forest bathing works was a big priority. Researchers had already been looking at markers of parasympathetic nerve activity such as blood pressure, heart rate, and heart rate variability. Cortisol, the stress hormone connected to much of the negative health effects of chronic stress, was easy to measure and likely part of the forest bathing picture.

In study after study, researchers found that forest bathers had lower measurements of cortisol than urban bathers. This cortisol-lowering effect of forest bathing was consistent in healthy adults, people with high blood pressure, and people with sleep disorders, depression, alcoholism, and even chronic pain. Across the board, forest bathing was lowering people's stress hormone levels. Researchers also determined that forest bathers' subjective experiences—that is, their own reports of how they felt—were in line with lower cortisol levels. Not only do forest bathers say they feel less stressed, the lab work shows that their bodies also feel less stressed and are making less stress hormone. Measurements of urinary adrenaline or noradrenaline, other hormones produced by the body during times of stress, also decreased after forest bathing. Similar studies have shown lower concentrations of cortisol as well as lower pulse rates, blood pressure, and heart rate variability, a measure of the variation in time between each heartbeat.

Cortisol is a great marker for stress, but nervous system activity can also be measured directly. Measurements of parasympathetic and sympathetic nerve activity show that the nervous system responds directly to its external environment. In stressful situations, sympathetic nerve activity is higher, while in calm, relaxed scenarios, parasympathetic nerve activity is higher. Much the way cortisol is lowered as a result of forest bathing, parasympathetic nerve activity is higher than sympathetic nerve activity while people are forest bathing. Likewise, parasympathetic nerve activity is lower than sympathetic nerve activity in city environments. These results confirm what most of us have already known to be true. Behind the scenes, your body is actually more relaxed in natural environments.

Research in Scotland shows the same effects as the forest bathing research done in Japan. Scottish researchers wondered if the impacts of green space differed among people of different socioeconomic status. Did forest bathing work only for the middle and upper classes? To answer this question, they looked at green space access in socioeconomically marginalized, urban communities. They discovered that the more green space there was close to where a person lived, the lower their cortisol and overall stress levels were, irrespective of their socioeconomic status and other financial stressors. Green space access doesn't make people more relaxed because wealthier middle- and upper-class neighborhoods have more green space. Green space access is an independent factor affecting health, separate from other social determinants.

Gender, however, might make a difference in the impact of forest bathing on stress. When researchers in Scotland broke the information down by gender, they found that women garnered more benefits than men. Cortisol, the critical stress hormone they measured in the study, normally goes up and down during the day and night in a relatively predictable curve. It is highest first thing in the morning, to help you get out of bed, and lowest overnight. In situations of chronic stress, cortisol patterns can become abnormal and unhealthy. During the forest bathing study, the women who went into the woods had healthier cortisol patterns compared with the women who spent their time in the city. These differences weren't found in the men who took part in this study.

GET HEALTHIER

Nature, time, and patience, are the three great physicians.
—*English proverb*

Nature is the best doctor. Forest bathing is good for your health. Whether or not you have an emotional or intrinsic connection to nature is irrelevant in terms of the potential for health benefits. Research has shown that forest bathing has positive effects on everything from high blood pressure to diabetes, dementia, and attention deficit hyperactivity disorder (ADHD). The amount of research looking into what forest bathing can do for your body is constantly growing and changing. It can be vast and overwhelming, much like the complex, multifaceted interactions we have with our larger ecosystem. While a lot of the research has been conducted in Japan, European researchers have also been studying the positive health effects of nature exposure. I've been distilling this research over the past decade, teaching other naturopathic, functional medicine, and integrative doctors in North America how to help our patients understand and reap the benefits of forest bathing and the healing power of nature. This section summarizes the most current research on forest bathing and nature exposure in general.

A note about the research available. Most of the research on forest bathing has focused on young and middle-aged Japanese men. A lot of the studies have been quite small, which makes them less reliable than studies with thousands or tens of thousands of participants. Few of the studies have been replicated, so it's hard to say whether they are accurate or reproducible, both of which are critical to authenticating the health benefits of forest bathing.

There are other reasons to take the current state of forest bathing research with a grain of salt. Most of the currently available research has looked at single sessions or a few daily sessions in a row. This short-term approach to research is in stark contrast with the nature of the health conditions that researchers are hoping to help through forest bathing. Health conditions such as high blood pressure, diabetes, heart disease, and mental illness are not short-term, acute problems with easy-fix solutions. They are chronic, complex conditions that require long-term solutions. To truly evaluate potential health benefits and effectiveness, forest bathing research needs to design long-term lifestyle-based studies that incorporate regular forest bathing sessions into the lives of participants.

Doctors almost never talk in absolutes. Nothing is for certain in medicine, scary as that is. Talking about forest bathing research is no different. Doctors and researchers overuse statements like "appears to" or "may be likely to." Without citing gold-standard, large-scale, high-quality systematic reviews or meta-analyses (where researchers pool data from several comparable, smaller studies to get the big picture), I'm likely to be criticized by some in the scientific community for what I've already said—that forest bathing is good for your health.

From a clinical research perspective, it's hard to write that forest bathing definitively does anything at all, since it doesn't fit neatly into the methodology of randomized controlled trials. Many studies compare forest bathing with city bathing without accounting for the seemingly endless factors that are hard to control, such as the weather. If the weather is different enough between the forest and the city, it's virtually impossible to determine whether an improvement in health may be attributed to the temperature or humidity or to the forest bathing experience itself. This is further complicated by the fact that forests and large parks often have lower temperatures than surrounding areas in a city. In the center of a large park at night, air temperatures can be up to 13 degrees Fahrenheit (7 degrees Celsius) cooler.

Nonetheless, I'll say it again. Forest bathing is good for your health. Like diet and exercise, nature exposure is one of the cornerstones to a healthy lifestyle. There are very few health risks in forest bathing and lots of potential benefits. Even if there is only one single meta-analysis with adequate proof of better health outcomes (hint: it's on blood pressure), I'll still be recommending it to my patients for a variety of reasons, from stress to mood disorders to dementia, insomnia, and more.

Live longer

Trees may be literally saving our lives. Even before we are born, our exposure to nature or lack of it is already impacting our health. Babies born closer to green spaces and under denser tree canopies are less likely to be born too small or too early. The denser the canopy, the higher the babies' birth weight and the less likely they are to be born small for gestational age or preterm. These effects are even more pronounced for babies born to parents who have had less postsecondary education and parents with lower incomes.

Access to nature can put people at an advantage before birth and throughout their entire life. Forests and parks help you live better, and they may even help you live longer. People who live in countries with more green space live longer than those who reside in countries with fewer natural resources. In Japan, people living in prefectures with the greatest amount of forest cover have the lowest rates of lung, breast, colon, uterine, prostate, and kidney cancers. In Shanghai, China, people living in the greenest neighborhoods have the lowest risk of overall mortality. In the United States, people living in green deserts, neighborhoods with the least green space as measured by satellites, are the most likely to die from a heart attack or stroke. The same associations have been found in the United Kingdom as well.

The closer you live to nature, the lower your risk of dying from any cause. People living within 0.62 miles (one kilometer) of green space have a lower chance of being diagnosed with coronary heart disease, neck pain, back pain, depression, anxiety, upper respiratory tract infections, asthma, chronic obstructive pulmonary disease (COPD), migraines, vertigo, gastrointestinal infections, urinary tract infections, diabetes, and medically unexplained physical symptoms.

The more trees in your city, the better. Having ten more trees per city block is like having a life expectancy improvement equivalent to a salary raise of $10,000 per year or being seven years younger. Walkable green streets in cities such as Tokyo may actually increase the longevity of seniors.

Even when accounting for affluence, the relationship between proximity to green space and longevity persists. People with low incomes and high nature proximity have mortality rates similar to those with higher socioeconomic status. People with low income and low nature proximity, however, have significantly higher rates of mortality. Rather than simply being a marker of wealth, green space is its own independent variable and a social determinant of health. Just as education, income, employment status, age, race/ethnicity, and social and community supports are all individual factors affecting health, nature exposure also impacts health on its own. How green your neighborhood is or isn't is one measure of your health equity.

Keep a healthy beat

Researchers have shown that forest bathing, the practice of sitting in the forest, lowers your blood pressure, pulse, and heart rate variability. Most of the studies done on forest bathing have measured blood pressure before and after forest bathing, often comparing it with blood pressure measurements before and after city or urban bathing. Although the results vary from one study to another, the trend is clear. Forest bathing lowers both systolic and diastolic blood pressure (the top and bottom numbers of your blood pressure reading, respectively). In this case, there's even a meta-analysis (the research equivalent of a definitive guide to x) that looked at blood pressure and forest bathing. Systolic blood pressure numbers are lower in people who already have high blood pressure (greater than 130 mm Hg before forest bathing) and also in people with healthy, normal blood pressure (less than 130 mm Hg). In people with high blood pressure, forest bathing lowers systolic blood pressure by around 6.33 mm Hg; in those with normal blood pressure, it lowers systolic blood pressure by around 3.85 mm Hg. Diastolic blood pressure, pulse rate, and heart rate are also lower after forest bathing compared with these measurements after city bathing.

These effects appear to be even more pronounced in middle-aged and older adults. The older you are, the more you get out of forest bathing. In a study in China, elderly adults diagnosed with hypertension experienced a reduction in blood pressure after forest bathing for seven days. A control group of similar adults walking in the city had no change in their blood pressure. Likewise, other markers of heart health (endothelin-1, homocysteine, and angiotensin II receptors) improved in the forest bathers but not in the city bathers. You might not be able to replace your blood pressure–lowering medication with forest bathing, but forest bathing is a low-risk way to reduce your blood pressure and work on heart disease prevention.

Prevention may be the key to understanding both the short- and long-term health effects of forest bathing. Coronary artery disease is the most common type of heart disease and the leading cause of death for both men and women. It happens when there is buildup of plaque on the inner walls of the arteries that feed the heart. Inflammation, hardening of the arteries, and narrowing of the blood vessels all happen in response. Like sludge in your sink drain, plaque can block the flow of blood, and thus oxygen, to the heart, leading to angina or a heart attack. Long-term, it can lead to other problems such as arrhythmia, irregular heart rhythms, and heart failure.

Since coronary artery disease is both common and fatal, doctors are constantly searching for ways to prevent it from getting worse or, better yet, from starting in the first place. Whenever I see a patient with a strong family history of heart disease (that includes mine), I recommend simple diet and lifestyle changes to help prevent plaque formation and inflammation. Regular exercise has always been a part of that overall strategy, but in the past few years, I've been more specific about where that exercise should take place—outdoors in nature.

Research on forest bathing has shown that where you exercise matters. In a study of people diagnosed with coronary artery disease, daily twenty-minute walks in a city park were more effective in lowering heart rates and diastolic blood pressure than walking on city streets. People who walked in the park were also able to walk longer and recover faster than city walkers. Walking in a park environment is better for heart function than walking in the city. This information is a game changer for everyone: from rehabilitation after a heart attack, to living with a heart condition, to long-term prevention.

Studies on heart failure and forest bathing are just as promising. Chronic heart failure (CHF), also known as congestive heart failure, is a common condition where the heart doesn't pump blood as well as it should. Around 6.5 million American adults have been diagnosed with heart failure. Related to other metabolic conditions such as high blood pressure, diabetes, and obesity, CHF can lead to shortness of breath, fatigue, and swelling. Studies on people with CHF have looked at measurements of brain natriuretic peptide (BNP) before and after forest bathing. BNP is a substance used to evaluate heart failure, because it increases when the heart is stretched and working hard to pump blood. After forest bathing, people with CHF show lower levels of BNP. These effects on BNP may be temporary, but more research is needed to show whether more frequent forest bathing might keep levels of BNP low and improve symptoms, quality of life, and other outcomes for people living with heart failure.

Forest bathing has also been shown to decrease stress hormone levels related to heart health. Two separate studies conducted in China compared the effects of spending a few nights in either a forest or a city environment on heart health in people diagnosed with CHF. In both studies, the results showed that exposure to the forest environment led to reductions in both oxidative stress and pro-inflammatory levels compared with staying in an urban environment. Serum cortisol levels (there's that stress link again) and the concentration of plasma endothelin-1, a vasoconstrictor peptide related to heart disease, were both significantly lower after forest bathing compared with the results after city bathing. One of the studies also measured angiotensin II type 2 receptors, which play a protective role in the development of CHF. In the forest group, angiotensin II type 2 receptors increased after forest bathing. No significant change was noted in the group that stayed in the city. These results are consistent with other studies looking at forest bathing and stress, mood, and overall measures of health.

Regulate your blood sugar

The health effects of forest bathing are generalized and affect lots of different body systems. Blood sugar regulation is just one of the metabolic effects of spending time in the woods. In one study on adults with type 2 diabetes, repetitive forest bathing sessions resulted in lower blood sugar readings. Although very few studies look at blood sugar, this particular study is important because it observed the long-term effects of forest bathing. Almost one hundred people participated in nine forest bathing sessions over six years. Not only did blood sugar significantly decrease immediately after each forest bathing session, but forest bathing showed lasting effects. At the end of the six years, the forest bathers had lower levels of hemoglobin A1c, a blood test that measures average blood sugar concentrations over the past two to three months, compared with their levels at the start of the study. The results documented the potential for forest bathing to improve insulin resistance and blood sugar regulation over the long haul.

A few studies also show that forest bathing might improve metabolism in a specific way that helps with weight loss. People with lower-than-normal levels of adiponectin, a hormone produced by fat cells, are at greater risk for diabetes, heart disease, obesity, and other metabolic conditions. However, two studies showed increases in the production of adiponectin in participants who had been forest bathing, compared with those in the control groups.

Kick-start your immune system

Forest bathing is like a natural boost to your immune system. Japanese forest bathing researchers knew from botanists, arborists, and other tree experts that the phytoncides in trees helped to protect the conifers from both disease and pests. Herbalists and other health care practitioners had been using conifer tree medicine, rich in those same volatile oils, to help humans fend off diseases caused by pests too. Usually, those volatile oils or the herbal medicines prepared from conifers had been taken internally or used topically. Although they were also used to support the immune system as inhalants, as in the case of steam inhalation to help clear nasal and breathing passages, little research had been done on the ability of phytoncides to work in humans just by sitting in the forest, a rather indirect application of their medicines.

Studies done in the lab showed that phytoncides released by trees could increase natural killer cells, a type of white blood cell critical in fighting off viruses and killing cancer cells. Human studies have confirmed both traditional knowledge and these in vitro results. After a couple of days of light walking in a forest, natural killer cell counts are consistently higher than they are when compared with their counts before the walk. Not only are natural killer cells increased, but other immune cells called T lymphocytes are boosted as well. It's not just about the numbers of immune cells either. The activity of those immune cells increases too. Measurements of chemicals released when natural killer cells attack show that forest bathing boosts overall immune function in ways that help you fend off illness and immune dysfunctions. Other studies have shown similar results—increases in natural killer cell counts and activity, in some cases lasting for up to thirty days after the forest bathing trip had ended.

Other kinds of immune cell responses show some evidence that forest bathing can decrease immune markers related to inflammation and autoimmune disease. Cytokines, proteins that act like chemical messengers, are often released by immune cells. Like a fire alarm or home security alarm, these cytokines light up and signal the body that a strong and fast reaction is needed. Two of these cytokines, TNFα (tumor necrosis factor alpha) and IL-6 (interleukin 6), can induce systemic inflammation through fevers, release of stress hormones, insulin resistance, acute phase reactants such as C-reactive protein (CRP), and appetite suppression. Locally, they are responsible for the cardinal signs of inflammation: heat, swelling, redness, and pain. They have been implicated in a variety of diseases, including rheumatoid arthritis, Alzheimer's, psoriasis, inflammatory bowel disease, and even depression. Unsurprisingly, both TNFα and IL-6, two markers of inflammation, are decreased after forest bathing sessions.

The importance of these studies, however, shouldn't be understated. Many of the immune markers studied in forest bathing research are connected to critical and common chronic health conditions, including cancer. A substantial amount of cancer research is directed toward investigating what adjunctive therapies might help to make chemotherapy and radiation treatments more effective by stimulating the body's immune system to help out in the process. Forest bathing may very well become a mainstay of those adjunctive therapies.

Sleep better

Being outdoors, and away from artificial light, helps synchronize your biology to natural circadian rhythms. Scientists investigating chronobiology, the study of biological rhythms, have shown that our connection to natural light/dark cycles helps to regulate our sleep, our moods, our stress levels, and our hormones.

As most of us know all too well, stress affects our sleep. We might have trouble falling asleep or staying asleep, and sometimes we may even end up feeling like we need more sleep and wake up groggy and struggle to get out of bed. Forest bathing researchers understood this connection between stress and sleep, so they looked at the impacts of forest bathing on sleep. What they found was consistent with their theories: people slept better and slept longer after forest bathing. Total sleep time was higher after a single forest bathing session. This is especially true for people who have a history of poor sleep. For example, people with insomnia and seniors with dementia get more sleep improvements out of forest bathing than people who are already great sleepers.

As an avid camper and a lifelong night owl, I know firsthand how this connection between forest bathing and better sleeping works. When you spend your day outside, you are constantly exposed to the outside air and sun. You witness the sun go up, usually waking with first light. And you witness the sun going down, because a sunset without buildings blocking your view is one of the most beautiful sights and you don't want to miss it. Once it gets dark enough, you look up to the night sky. With less light pollution blocking your view, you get to see the stars and you can look at constellations that you haven't seen living in the city. If the conditions are just right, you might actually see the Milky Way or a meteor shower. And then you pass out.

Outdoors, even without doing more exercise than you would at home, your body becomes attuned to the natural light and dark cycles throughout the day. You harmonize with nature's rhythms and cycles. The sun sends you a message through sunlight during the day, and since you're outside, you can receive it. Sunlight hits your skin and eyes while you are awake and tells your body what to do when the lights go out. Once the sun goes down, your body starts up the sleep program. It releases the hormone melatonin, which triggers sleepiness and then signals the release of other dark-loving hormones such as growth hormone. (P.S. Your mama was right. You do grow in your sleep.)

Think and work better

In children, time spent in natural settings decreases ADHD symptoms. In adults, contact with nature improves focus, concentration, and work productivity. Scandinavian research shows that employees with the greatest degree of nature exposure perform better and are more dedicated to and engaged in their work. They express less cynicism and experience less professional burnout too.

Walking in a park setting or forest bathing increases all executive functions, the set of skills critical to planning, organizing, and completing tasks. Nature exposure helps us keep track of what we're doing and get things done more effectively and efficiently. Looking at nature scenes can enhance accuracy and speed up reaction times. Memory recall is also boosted by forest bathing. In people diagnosed with major depressive disorder, memory is often affected, either by the depression itself or sometimes as an unfortunate side effect of antidepressant medications. After a forest bathing session, people with depression performed better on memory tasks than they did after urban walking.

Forest bathing and other nature activities help our brains work better in the moment and over the long run. Avid, daily gardeners over sixty-five years old who don't have any cognitive impairments are 35 percent less likely to develop dementia over the next fifteen years of their lives compared with seniors who rarely garden. Nature exposure with some physical activity, such as the act of gardening, can be a great way to prevent age-related cognitive impairments.

Not only are garden exposure and active gardening a great way to prevent dementia, they are an effective part of an overall approach to the treatment of dementia as well. Dementia is pervasive nowadays, affecting close to fifty million people worldwide. Although there are pharmaceutical options that can help slow down or minimize progression, there is currently no known therapy or treatment that can lead to a cure. Living with dementia can be frustrating, as people find themselves increasingly less capable of expressing their needs and feelings because of cognitive impairments beyond their control. In later stages of the disease, especially in cases where people with dementia need the support of a live-in home care provider or long-term-care environment, frustrations can lead to agitation and other behaviors that can easily be misinterpreted as anxiety, depression, and/or aggression. The good news is that people with dementia who have access to therapeutic gardens and outdoor spaces exhibit fewer of these types of behaviors.

Research has compared gardening activities with other types of activities such as puzzles, collaging, and origami in patients with dementia. After six weeks of either gardening or art activities, the people who spent thirty minutes a day outside in the garden were less agitated and aggressive than the people who spent the same amount of time doing art projects.

People with dementia who spend time in a garden, indoors or out, regardless of what they do during that time, have better quality of life overall. Whether they plant seeds, water plants, or just sit in a garden, patients with dementia who interact with nature are less agitated throughout the day and perform better on cognitive tests. They spend less time pacing and exhibit fewer violent and escape-seeking behaviors. Garden time also improves social interaction time for patients living with dementia in residential facilities with their visitors and with staff. They are more actively engaged with other people and show more sustained attention while visiting with family members and doing other activities.

The health benefits extend well beyond cognitive tests and behaviors too. People with dementia sleep better and longer and feel more rested when they wake up. Those who spend time in gardens are prescribed lower doses of antipsychotics, likely as a result of positive behavioral changes. Since antipsychotic medications are related to an increased risk of falls, the total number of falls and the severity of falls also decrease after garden time is implemented for people living with dementia. The positive domino-like health effects of gardening quickly add up for patients with dementia. According to their nurses, doctors, and family members, people living with dementia who have access to a garden experience better quality of life overall than they did when they lived somewhere without garden access.

Balance your mood

Ever notice how you feel better when you're looking out the window or spending time outside in nature? Does your mood shift, depending on where you are? It may seem like common sense, but it's actually true and there is plenty of science to back it up. Where you live impacts your mood. Rates of mental illness are higher in urban centers than in rural areas. Urban dwellers are more likely to be diagnosed with depression, anxiety, and schizophrenia. Even within cities, people who live closer to green space tend to have better mental health. If you live close to a city park, you are less likely to struggle with anxiety and depression. Even folks who are less socially connected to other people feel better if they live closer to nature. In clinical terms, nature exposure is associated with greater subjective well-being, satisfying a need for connection in people who feel socially isolated.

Looking at nature makes us feel better, even if it's from a window. Our mental well-being is better, even momentarily, if we can see trees, see or hear water, hear birds singing, or feel in contact with nature. Using a cell phone app, researchers track users' mental well-being in different kinds of spaces using a quick series of questions and a photo taken using their phones. They found that people rated their mental well-being significantly higher if they were outdoors or if they could see trees or hear birds. These mental health benefits were particularly enhanced in people who displayed impulsivity, a personality trait associated with ADHD, addiction, and schizophrenia.

Walking in nature has been shown to improve mood and short-term memory in people with depression, as well as decrease rumination (repetitive, negative thoughts) and brain activity associated with mental illness. Several forest bathing studies show significant decreases in anxiety levels as measured on standardized scales such as the State-Trait Anxiety Inventory. In forest bathing studies, these mood-lifting effects are more pronounced in people who have been diagnosed with depression, people living with chronic fatigue syndrome, and those who have been diagnosed with alcohol abuse and addiction. Nature exposure is good for your mood, all the more so if you're already feeling down.

People who participate in research studies consistently say that they feel more relaxed, comfortable, and attentive after forest bathing. In general, forest bathers answering survey questions feel more positive. Their affect and mood ameliorate, and their scores on standardized tests such as the Beck Depression Inventory match those improvements. They feel more vigor, vitality, and liveliness. People with chronic pain and depression experience reductions in both after forest bathing and have improvements in their health-related quality of life. Even people with cancer who had recently finished surgical, chemotherapeutic, or radiation treatment express a greater sense of emotional well-being and self-realization after forest bathing.

Early spring can be a difficult time for many people with depression. Especially for those with seasonal affective disorder, where the lack of light and outdoor time and vitamin D conspires to dampen their moods, spring doesn't usually promote an immediate lift. It can feel as though everyone else around you is ecstatic while you still feel like crap. In fact, rates of suicide are highest in midspring (May in the Northern Hemisphere and November in the Southern Hemisphere), just as the seasons change. Although there is some debate as to why suicide rates are higher in spring, the fact remains that spring is often a time when people with depression need more support. Regular forest bathing sessions during this period can be an effective addition to comprehensive strategies to bridge the seasonal risk.

One of my patients came to me specifically to try to prevent this worsening of suicidal thoughts and urges during the spring that she had been experiencing for fifteen years. She didn't have seasonal allergies, which have been theorized to play a role, but she did notice that she felt her energy increase before her mood. As with many people, this increase in energy without a concurrent shift in mood can seem to act on suicidal thoughts. Together with her psychotherapist, I worked out a plan for her to adopt starting in March to set up a smoother spring.

One of the critical pieces was daily forest bathing in the park near her home. She didn't feel she had enough energy for full-blown exercise, which in general is great for depression, but she could manage to walk to the park and sit on a bench under the trees for fifteen to twenty minutes. While she was there, she would listen to a guided meditation to help avoid any tendencies toward negative self-talk, ruminating, and catastrophizing. After one week, she reported that she had fewer urges to self-harm, and when she did have those thoughts, they seemed to last five to ten minutes instead of what seemed like hours. After two weeks of regular forest bathing, she was able to walk around the park and get gentle exercise. By mid-April, she had been forest bathing for over a month and noticed that she hadn't needed to visit her medical doctor for an increased dosage of her antidepressant medication. She had her ups and downs but overall felt that the passage into spring was more bearable than in past years. She continued with regular forest bathing through the summer and fall, although down to three or four days a week. Her mood stayed stable and her sense of self improved.

Forest bathing helps you feel better about yourself and how you look too. Both looking at pictures of natural versus built environments and going on forest bathing walks compared with city bathing walks led to better body image and self-appreciation in four separate studies with university students. Engagement with nature in other studies also points to higher self-esteem, self-compassion, and body appreciation.

After forest bathing, people tend to become more patient and feel that they have more self-control. Overreactions and aggression are less likely responses to irritation, even when provoked. One fascinating study looked at how aggressive people became during a competitive game when it was played in a natural location and then in an urban one. Even when tired and depleted and instigated by their opponent honking a loud horn, people in the natural environments responded less aggressively than people in the urban locations. Correctional officers involved in an experimental study at an institution in Oregon noted that inmates in solitary confinement who exercised in a room that played nature videos displayed calmer behavior than solitary confinement inmates who worked out in a gym without any videos. In a way, nature exposure makes us better people.

If you're seeing a psychotherapist as part of your overall approach to mental health, it's probably worth asking about nature-based psychotherapy. Cognitive-behavioral therapy conducted in an arboretum was more effective in reducing symptoms of depression and resulting in complete remission than the same therapy offered in a hospital setting. The setting for psychotherapy, it appears, can help to boost the effects of therapy and become part of therapy itself. It's a huge part of the reason I've been offering naturopathic appointments outside in my office garden. Why not take advantage of the space and take a two-for-one approach to health?

Forest bathing combined with exercise itself is also good for overall mental health and seems to be even better than either one alone. Green exercise can improve mood and self-esteem. Studies comparing forest bathing and walking with walking in an urban environment have shown that green exercise significantly decreases feelings of tension, anxiety, depression, dejection, anger, hostility, fatigue, and confusion.

Researchers haven't yet determined exactly why people feel better outside, but some studies have hinted at possible mechanisms. Levels of dopamine, a neurotransmitter involved in depression, anxiety, and compulsive behaviors such as addictions, appear to be lower after forest bathing. Likewise, levels of adrenaline and noradrenaline, two of the neurotransmitters responsible for the fight-or-flight response, are also lower after forest bathing. Like mindful meditation, yoga, and exercise, forest bathing appears to decrease sympathetic nerve activity and activate parasympathetic nerve activity.

Brain scans of people during forest bathing sessions offer an explanation into why nature makes us happy. A specific area of the brain called the "subgenual prefrontal cortex" is most active when people are ruminating, replaying the same negative feeling or worrying about the same thing over and over again. When someone is engaging in any kind of negative self-talk, this particular part of the prefrontal cortex lights up. When researchers compared forest bathers with urban walkers, not only did the forest bathers say that their mood had improved, but their subgenual prefrontal cortices were less active. Forest bathing can help us to ruminate less often, engage in less negative self-talk, and make space for positive mental health states and greater self-compassion.

Other studies of brain waves show similar effects. Electroencephalography analyses measuring electrical brain activity show increases in high alpha wave activity with forest bathing. Alpha waves are most active when we feel alert and calm at the same time. They are associated with mental relaxation and feelings of euphoria. In contrast, lower alpha waves, related to fear and sadness, are found with city bathing. Beta wave activity seems to follow a similar pattern. Forest bathing increases beta waves, while city bathing decreases them. Increased beta waves are associated with attentiveness, especially in task-oriented activities such as decision making and problem solving. Like other markers in forest bathing research studies, these results are similar to results in research studies on meditation and relaxation techniques.

Breathe easier

Air pollution is a growing problem many cities are facing. It's common knowledge that trees make for less polluted environments. Forests help clean up the air by converting carbon dioxide into oxygen and releasing that oxygen back into the environment. Carbon dioxide is the worst offender when it comes to climate change, but it isn't the main health risk in terms of air pollution. The biggest health offender in air pollution is particulate matter, microscopic particles that get trapped in our lungs when we breathe polluted air.

Particulate matter is estimated to cause 3.2 million deaths per year, primarily from stroke and heart attacks. Trees clean the air by directly absorbing particulate matter or trapping the particles on the surface of their leaves. The Nature Conservancy estimates that the average tree can absorb anywhere from 7 to 24 percent of the particulate matter in its vicinity. Simply put, more trees equal cleaner air.

There is some nuance, however, to where trees should be planted to make their air-cleaning effects most effective. At least in cities, trees planted too close together can actually trap pollutants under the canopy, in effect increasing air pollution exposure by impeding air flow. We shouldn't blame the trees, however. This problem exists only in places where there are already lots of tall buildings stopping the natural air flow currents in addition to heavy traffic flow of diesel- and gas-powered vehicles. Perhaps we shouldn't plant trees just anywhere, but we should still be planting them.

Overall, less pollution equals cleaner air. Clean air makes it easier to breathe for people with asthma and other respiratory health conditions, including emphysema and chronic bronchitis. Many people with breathing problems already know that they feel better when they spend time outside the city in a more rural area. Many of them already know that forest bathing is good for them. Research is starting to catch up to what people have long known: forest bathing equals easier breathing. Forest bathing can decrease exposure to air pollutants, lower airway inflammation, and reduce stress, a known trigger for acute breathing problems in people with asthma and COPD (chronic obstructive pulmonary disease).

Research shows that elderly adults with COPD experience health benefits from forest bathing. COPD is a chronic, inflammatory lung disease that makes it hard to breathe. There are two types of COPD—chronic bronchitis with a mucous cough; and emphysema, where there is also damage to lung tissue. The disease progression of COPD involves several factors, one of which is cell death caused by white blood cells that express certain chemicals known as perforin and granzyme B. Other inflammatory markers such as IL-6, IL-8, CRP, and TNFα are also involved whenever someone with COPD has an acute exacerbation. In one forest bathing study, perforin inside white blood cells was lower after forest bathing compared with its level after city bathing. IL-6, IL-8, CRP, and TNFα were also lower with forest bathing but not with city bathing. These same inflammatory markers that decrease with forest bathing are also lowered by corticosteroids, the standard treatment for COPD. Stress markers such as cortisol and epinephrine were also reduced in the forest bathing group.

Healthy kids

Getting kids to spend time outside has positive effects on their psychological and emotional development. Forest bathing helps children increase their physical activity levels, improve their eyesight, lower the chance that they'll be overweight, improve their behavior, and reduce symptoms associated with ADHD. Forest bathing also fosters positive environmental attitudes and values. Children (and adults too!) learn to conserve, protect, and live harmoniously with their larger environment, making them better stewards for the future of our planet. As Philippe Cousteau Sr., cinematographer and son of Jacques Cousteau, said: "People can only protect what they love, but they can only love what they know."

When children practice forest bathing, they develop their powers of observation. Children can learn to use their "owl eyes" to notice things with their peripheral vision or crouch low to the ground to watch a caterpillar crawl over a leaf. They get accustomed to using their "bat ears" and learn to become quiet to listen to the birds sing or to hear the sound of a woodpecker. Kids learn to focus in nature and pay attention to the natural world.

Outside in nature, children's play becomes more imaginative. A stick or a leaf can become anything. Learning becomes more imaginative too. While playing outside, kids develop skills across multiple learning domains, from math and biology to engineering and social studies. Kids playing in nature work better in teams and develop more cooperative and collaborative relationships with peers, skills that are needed later in the workplace. Forest bathing for kids encourages both autonomy and empathy, which in turn is related to decreases in aggressive behavior.

Being outside encourages free play, exploration, leisure, and child-initiated learning. It improves coordination, balance, and agility as children move on uneven ground. I can vividly remember the first few times I took my children hiking on a natural dirt trail, and especially when we went backcountry canoe camping for the first time. Toddlers are already unstable on their feet. At first, it seemed as though they were tripping over everything. It took some time before they were able to walk over or around the tree roots and pebbles and pinecones that create the textured forest floor, but now they bounce with ease down any dirt path. It takes much more balance and concentration and responsiveness than putting one foot in front of the other without paying attention on a concrete sidewalk. Learning to pay attention and focus may be why kids who spend less time in green spaces are more likely to show signs of ADHD, but it isn't the whole story about the benefits of children getting outside.

Kids who live near green spaces are more likely to spend time outside and get enough physical activity. In New York, preschool children from lower-income families are less likely to be overweight or obese if they live in a neighborhood with greater tree density. The same has been found in studies of children in other cities.

How much and what kind of greenery children can see from their schoolrooms may impact how well they perform academically. Studies of public schools in Michigan found that kids who had greener views from their classrooms and cafeterias scored better on standardized assessments, even after controlling for other known factors affecting kids' grades such as class size and socioeconomic status. Seeing trees and shrubs (rather than grass or playing fields) from their windows also increased the likelihood those kids would graduate from high school and would apply for university programs.

UNPLUG

In all natural things there is somewhat of the marvellous.

—*Aristotle*

You've probably seen that meme that has been circulated for the past few years with a picture in the forest that reads: "There is no Wi-Fi in the forest, but I promise that you'll find a better connection." It's a catchy phrase and I appreciate the ethos of the saying, but it isn't accurate. The problem is, the truth isn't quite as catchy and doesn't make for a good meme. Reality check: More than likely there *is* Wi-Fi in the forest, but I promise if you put down your phone, you'll find a different kind of connection.

Not everyone means the same thing when they say they are going to unplug. Very few people are looking for somewhere there is absolutely no cell service as a feature of forest bathing. In fact, upward of 97 percent of campers say they are bringing their smartphones or other digital devices with them to campgrounds.

Unplugging doesn't even mean that you can't bring your smartphone. Even on backcountry canoe camping trips, I'll often bring a phone for safety reasons but not necessarily turn it on. Unplugging can mean staying off social media and just using your phone to take pictures and then waiting to post until you get home. It might mean using your phone for apps and information. For some, it means not checking notifications or reading work emails as they come in. For others, having access to Wi-Fi or cellular service means they can actually spend more time outdoors than they would otherwise. Being able to check or send the odd work email can actually increase access to and opportunities for forest bathing for some people who wouldn't otherwise be able to.

The benefits of unplugging is also about putting your phone down and looking at things at a distance. Looking far away is good for our brains and our eyes. Staring at a screen is the new normal. Most of us spend most of our days connected to some sort of screen. If we aren't using a computer for work, we're staring at our tablets and smartphones. Digital technology is everywhere and digital eye strain is on the rise.

A few years ago, when I celebrated my fortieth birthday, I joked with my optometrist that I was on my way to bifocals. After my eye exam, she joked with me. "You don't need bifocals," she said, "but you did develop an astigmatism in your old age." I asked her how it happened and what I could do about it. "It's the same way you end up with bifocals," she told me. "You're spending too much time in front of a computer." Her solution: Stop staring at a screen for hours on end and take more breaks. The last time we were there with my kids, they too asked her how they could avoid needing glasses, since they have terrible genes on this front. She told them about the "20-20-20" rule. Every twenty minutes, look at something twenty feet away for twenty seconds.

Unplugging also comes back around to other aspects of our health like sleep. Our phones are a major source of blue light in our lives, especially in the evening and at night before bed. Blue light sends signals from our eyes through the optic nerves to the brain to let us know that it is daytime and we should be awake. In natural settings without technological sources of light, our bodies naturally shift into darkness alongside the rest of nature. Our circadian rhythm, or biological clock, is in tune with the sun and we make melatonin, the hormone that triggers sleepiness. When we use our phones or tablets or other sources of blue light in the evening and nighttime, our circadian rhythm gets out of sync.

My solution: Use your smartphone as a camera, but wait to post to social media until you have finished your forest bathing session. Spend more time using your eyes and your memory than your camera to capture the beauty of your forest bathing experience. Put your phone away in a zipped pocket or inside your backpack. Use technology as a way to help you get to nature or get to know it better. Use an app to track your time or activity in the forest in the background. Don't use your phone outside (or inside, for that matter) at night when your eyes could adjust to the darkness and maybe, just maybe, see the stars.

Don't be fooled—if you want to get the most benefits of being in nature, you need to leave those headphones at home. True forest bathing requires the use of all five senses. Unplug from your screen and plug into the forest.

BE MORE MINDFUL

Look deep, deep into nature, and then you will understand everything better.

—*Albert Einstein*

It's hard to be still and mindful in our world today. We are connected twenty-four hours a day to technology, between our computers, tablets, smartphones, and now wearables that track us even while we sleep. Culture encourages us to be busy, be productive, and be efficient. We try to multitask. We spend more time thinking about the past and the future than we do thinking about the present. Rather than focusing on the taste of our food and the act of chewing it, many of us are reading our Facebook or Instagram feeds while we're eating. Sometimes it's technology that distracts us. Other times it's our own thoughts that derail us from living in the moment. Being present in the moment isn't easy. Concepts like FOMO, the fear of missing out, remind us of our anticipation of things that may or may not happen at some undetermined time in the future. We struggle to find a way to just be.

Inspired by Buddhist and Shinto practices, forest bathing naturally has psychological and spiritual benefits. It can be a meditative or spiritual exercise. It engages you in nondirected attention and mindfulness meditation. Forest bathing instills a sense of peace and being at one with the world. It nurtures instinctive feelings of continuity with nature and overall life satisfaction. Personal and spiritual growth often come out of situations where we are filled with wonder and awe. They can also happen when we are quiet and able to listen to our inner wisdom or more easily access intuition.

Forest bathing can be a great introduction to the concept of transcendence. The practice of forest bathing naturally reminds us that there is something that exists beyond our self. Looking over the forest or through the seemingly endless thick of trees, we get a sense of the infinite possibilities in life. Forest bathing practice helps you to open your senses to nature, which helps you develop intuition. As you practice forest bathing more frequently, you become more receptive, reflective, and reflexive, allowing for increased self-awareness and personal growth.

Conceptually, forest bathing can also lead you into what psychologists call a "liminal space." Liminal means threshold, and a liminal space is a place of transition between what is known and infinite possibility, where you have let go of old ways of understanding or being or an old identity but don't yet anticipate what is coming next. Liminal space is ambiguous. It invites trust that answers will come, that a new path will emerge, or that you can change. Forest bathing, through mindfulness and nondirection (you don't have any goal in mind or end point, you don't even have to move your feet), can help create a space where you lose track of time and open yourself up to nascent and transformative experiences.

Forest bathing, like many experiences in nature, can be rather emotional and even spiritual. It isn't unusual for people deeply engaged in forest bathing to feel as though they have lost themselves as they sense a oneness with their environment. Being completely absorbed in the experience can lend itself to feelings of integration, consciousness, and a different kind of knowing.

One of my favorite day hikes near my home is along the Niagara Escarpment, a long cuesta or ridge that extends from New York through Ontario, Michigan, Wisconsin, and Illinois. The Niagara Escarpment is most famous for the cliff that the Niagara River plunges over, resulting in the gorgeous Niagara Falls. There are a multitude of trail options along the escarpment, including the Bruce Trail, which is the oldest and longest marked trail in Canada. I haven't had the opportunity to hike the entirety of its 550-mile (890-kilometer) length just yet, but I have spent a lot of time in contemplation along its route. I often find myself sitting on a rocky precipice, nestled against the trunk of a tree, staring off across the valley below. If I sit there long enough without interruption, I inevitably start to feel different. I feel a oneness with the natural world around me, as though I am a part of the larger whole, not separate looking at nature but rather looking out from within nature. The dirt, the forest, the cliffside, the trees, plants, moss, all feel like part of me, held together by a web of sorts (or perhaps fungi). It's hard to explain this sensation to someone who hasn't shared in this experience. It's almost like a religious experience to say that you feel a mountain or a river. The immensity and intensity of nature can be overwhelming, and invigorating, and perhaps even bring you closer to a sense of how small and yet so big you are within the wider natural world.

Astronaut Mae Jemison said it well in a 2005 CNN interview: "Once I got into space, I was feeling very comfortable in the universe. I felt like I had a right to be anywhere in this universe, that I belonged here as much as any speck of stardust, any comet, any planet." Although Jemison was talking about her experience aboard the flight deck on the space shuttle

Endeavor looking back at Chicago, she described an experience similar to sitting atop a mountain, or looking out across the ocean, or peering in between the trunks of trees through a seemingly endless forest. Jemison lays bare the deep connections we have with nature and the fact that we belong in nature, that we are indeed part of something much greater than ourselves.

TAKE A STAND

In nature, nothing is perfect and everything is perfect. Trees can
be contorted, bent in weird ways, and they're still beautiful.

—*Alice Walker*

Trees are great mentors for setting down roots and standing tall. Sometimes, taking a stand may be about living in your own authenticity, accepting yourself for, rather than in spite of, all your blemishes and imperfections. Loving the way your body twists and curves and still reaches for the sky. Other times, taking a stand is about standing tall in your beliefs and personal boundaries, waving with the wind yet remaining unwavering. It may mean heading straight for your goals, the way the conifer trees tend to grow their trunks straight toward the light in the sky.

Often, my patients come to me with unexplainable symptoms. They have already seen countless doctors for their mysterious ills and are still feeling afflicted in spite of an endless series of tests and treatments. Or sometimes they come directly to my door with a certainty that their physical symptoms are related to a specific stressor or trauma from their past. In one of these cases,

I had a patient come to see me for loss. She'd very recently lost a sibling to a heart attack and her grief was debilitating. She wanted to go help care for her nieces as they adjusted to a new life without their mother, but she could barely get out of bed. We talked at length about the feeling of shock she had and about tending to her own grief before holding space for other people's feelings. As she had been away from home when receiving the news about her sister's death, she had taken a plane home and was feeling ungrounded, as though she were stuck in the air in a space of transition. When I asked her about a place that felt grounded and safe, she immediately brought up the image of an elm tree that grew outside her childhood home. It occupied the view outside her bedroom window when she was growing up. She was able to imagine herself with that tree and felt her back against its trunk, gathering strength and comfort from its presence. The next day, she felt strong enough to drive to the home of her sister, who had lived near the house they grew up in, and spent time with that elm tree in person. She sent me pictures of the tree, noting how her grief had evolved from feelings of shock and paralysis to more manageable feelings of sadness and loss.

Trees can help us develop positive self-image and self-esteem, and they can also teach us about our place in community, guiding us to live more harmoniously with others. A stand of trees is imprecisely defined as a contiguous community with similar characteristics that distinguish them from another group of trees. A forest is merely a collection of stands. These distinctions may be most useful to forest managers and forestry departments, but they also have importance in forest bathing. A stand of trees and the larger forest of multiple stands are layers of community. They mirror our neighborhoods and cities and regions in their relationships with one another. Stands can give us insight into how to live with our relatives, codified in family trees. They can also guide us to more mutually beneficial interactions with our neighbors.

One tree is not a forest. It is the interdependence among trees and plants and animals that makes up a community. That community is the forest. A single tree on its own cannot withstand the stressors of wind or rain or snowstorms. Together, a forest can thrive. To work in concert with one another, trees have to communicate. Trees communicate with their neighbors through scent signals. Each tree can release chemical scents to warn its neighbors and to call helpful animals to eat predatory insects. Trees release these scent signals into the air, but they also communicate using chemicals released through their roots, traveling through the soil with the assistance of fungal networks. Dr. Suzanne Simard, a scientist researching tree communication, called these networks "the wood wide web."

Before they can use these fungal networks, trees must connect with them. Individual trees allow fungi to grow into the soft hairs on the tree's roots and connect to fungi and other trees, even different species of trees, through the forest floor. Fungal webs, known as mycelium, can grow for more than two thousand years and cover two thousand acres. These large networks help connect trees from one end of a forest to another, allowing for water and nutrient distribution as well as communication.

No tree represents this vision of community more completely than the trembling aspen, *Populus tremuloides*. Trembling aspen trees often grow in large colonies, and they are quick to establish themselves on disturbed soils. The remarkable thing about trembling aspens is that each tree is not in fact a unique, individual tree. What we perceive as a single trembling aspen tree is actually a clone of every other aspen in that stand. As old trunks die, the trembling aspen colony sends up a trunk that is precisely the same as every other shoot. Not only are these trees connected through the fungal network, they are also connected to one another through the colony's root system, each one an identical copy of the original trembling aspen tree. Individual colonies of trembling aspen are older than the oldest of trees. One colony in Utah is estimated to be more than eighty thousand years old, which makes it the oldest living organism on earth.

Humans create communities among people for the same reasons as trees. Together, we are stronger. Then, when we interact with trees, we become part of that interdependence too. The National Healing Forest Initiative is an organization that interweaves forest bathing with reconciliation between Indigenous and non-Indigenous communities in Canada. Communities and individuals are invited to create green spaces dedicated to healing the wounds associated with residential schools, missing and murdered Indigenous women, and the history of the Sixties Scoop (the practice of removing Indigenous children from their families and placing them in foster homes or putting them up for adoption). The healing forests in this network are intended for healing communities, building respect, and effecting social change as much as they are about the health of the individuals who might visit these spaces. They are an inspiring example of how, standing with trees, we can become stronger, healthier, and more connected.

GET INSPIRED

Study nature, love nature, stay close to nature. It will never fail
you.

—*Frank Lloyd Wright*

If you want to be creative, connect with creation. Nature has inspired authors such as Henry David Thoreau, Toni Morrison, and
Jack Kerouac, as well as painters such as Vincent van Gogh, Georgia O'Keeffe, and the Group of Seven. The American poet Joyce
Kilmer declared, "I think I shall never see, a poem lovely as a
tree." Playwright, performer, and activist Eve Ensler has written
about how a tree saved her life.

It's hard to imagine stories such as *Winnie-the-Pooh*, "Robin
Hood," "Snow White," or *The Wind in the Willows* without their
ever-present backdrop of the forest. Fairy tales and other fictional
stories in print and on-screen often refer to the magic and mystery of enchanted woods. Books such as Dr. Seuss's *The Lorax*,
Hayao Miyazaki's film *Princess Mononoke*, and James Cameron's
movie *Avatar* all center on the theme of protecting the soul or the
spirit of the forest.

Not everything inspired by nature shows only the bright side
of the forest. Folk stories such as "Baba Yaga," "Hansel and Gre-
tel," and "Little Red Riding Hood" warn children of the dark side
of the forest too. The forest outside Hogwarts in J. K. Rowling's
Harry Potter series has its dangers as well. This dark side of the
forest can be scary, but it is also where we find strength to face
our fears and grow into new versions of ourselves.

Today's authors and artists continue to go to the forest,

retreating to the woods for quiet inspiration and concentrated writing time. Although artist retreats may seem like nothing more than an extended working holiday, research supports the idea that forests evoke creativity. In one study, people improved their creativity scores by 50 percent after three days in nature. Being immersed in a safe, natural environment elicits a gentle, soft fascination with the things around you. Even though there is an abundance of sensory stimuli, forest bathing is a low-arousal activity, a level of engagement that is believed to be close to the "default mode" network of brain activity. This emotional and cognitive state allows for more restful introspection and then more creativity as a result. It's a long-winded way of saying that low levels of stimulation are the backbone of creativity. In the words of my children, being bored forces you to make up stories.

The forest has been an inspiration for authors and visual artists, and increasingly, artists are finding a home for their works within the forest setting too. There are more and more opportunities to forest bathe in an outdoor art gallery. Sculpture gardens have long provided an opportunity for art to be created that has its home outdoors, and today's artists continue to deliver and evolve this tradition. In Japan, the Kirishima Art Forest, encompassing thirty-two acres, includes a 1.24-mile (two-kilometer) garden trail with outdoor site-specific exhibitions enveloped in nature. American glass artist Dale Chihuly has frequently presented his glass sculptures in gardens and natural settings, reimagining the forest in magnificent shapes and colors. Sound artists have also moved into the woods, creating immersive sound installations, such as British artist Pete M. Wyer's iForest in the Adirondacks. The music "I Walk Towards Myself" was created for the specific site and land on which the twenty-four speakers are now hidden among the trees as visitors walk along a path and take in the music.

Some artists not only find inspiration from nature but actually manipulate nature into works of art. Artists working in this style create what is referred to as "land art" or "environmental art" by using the materials in front of them in nature. Robert Smithson's *Spiral Jetty* (1970), an arrangement of rocks, earth, and algae forming a jetty that juts out into the Great Salt Lake in Utah, is one of the more famous examples of land art. Forests and trees have played an important role too. Artist Joseph Beuys's *7000 Eichen* (1982) project involved Beuys and a group of volunteers planting seven thousand oak trees in Kassel, Germany, in artistic response to increasing urbanization. Other artists have created architecture out of willow trees and saplings, such as Patrick Dougherty's woven and tangled giant "stickworks" that resemble human-sized nests and cocoons.

We often look to trees for inspiration, as well as for advice on how to make sense of our lives. The forest is the literal home of mysticism, mythology, and religion around the world. In many cultures, forests and trees are the homes of nature deities and mythical creatures such as faeries, dryads, unicorns, elves, and ents. Other times, trees are the symbolic representation of a story, a belief, or even a door to another universe or another time.

The Tree of Life is one such example. An archetype of a sacred tree, it represents concepts such as immortality, connections between heaven and earth, fertility, and knowledge. Variations of the Tree of Life feature prominently in many different religions and times, from ancient Mesopotamia to the kabbalah to the Garden of Eden and the Koran. Mythical trees of life also feature prominently in the cosmologies of the Indigenous peoples of North America and Mesoamerica.

After I finished my undergraduate degree, I traveled through Central America. I visited cities and museums, and I learned Spanish. I hiked to hidden waterfalls and Mayan temples deep in the jungle. Quickly, I became fascinated with one tree in particular that I saw on my hikes, the ceiba (*Ceiba pentandra*). It had huge buttress roots that extended like ridges towering above the ground, a wide trunk, and a canopy so high that it seemed as though it might actually reach the sky. I immediately felt a sense of awe in its presence as I nestled into one of the coves created by the buttress roots. Even in an unknown forest, the little nook of the tree roots provided a feeling of safety from which I could just rest and observe the jungle before continuing on a walk.

Ceiba trees along hiking routes quickly became my preferred rest points. They often served as a marker along a trail but also as a place from which I would just watch and listen to nature. Underneath a ceiba tree, I could immerse myself in the forest, no matter how foreign or potentially unknown the environment was. Years later, I ran into the ceiba again on a trail in Costa Rica eponymously named *Sendero La Ceiba*. On that trail, a giant ceiba marked the halfway point on a hike through the rain forest that led to a field of lava rocks from an old eruption. My children, preschoolers at the time, needed a place to rest and to celebrate their achievement of having walked so far on their own.

I didn't know at the time that this powerful tree, the ceiba, was an integral part of Mayan cosmology and culture. The ceiba, in Mayan culture, symbolizes an axis mundi, a central world tree that serves as a connection point between heaven, earth, and the underworld. When I asked local friends about the ceiba tree, they told me that it was believed to extend seven planes into heaven and seven planes into the underworld as well. It's no wonder that the ceiba is the national tree of Guatemala.

FOREST ESSENCES

Trees are poems the earth writes upon the sky.

—*Khalil Gibran*

The essence of the forest is etched in my mind. The scents of pine, cedar, fir, and spruce trees bathe me in comfort and cleanse my spirit. They freshen the mind, clarify thoughts. The memories of smells take root in the limbic system in the brain, the same area responsible for holding emotions related to past events. That's why you can conjure up the memories of smells so easily. It even explains why some people might smell the forest when they visualize it or look at a picture of trees. If you've spent a lot of time in forest environments, you may even be bringing those smells to mind right now.

All these glorious smells are the result of volatile oils, so called because they evaporate easily into the air, wafting between the trees. The bulk of volatile oils are actually compounds called "terpenes," members of the largest class of naturally occurring organic compounds. Terpenes get further subdivided into monoterpenes, sesquiterpenes, and diterpenes. Distilled and concentrated into little vials, they are sold as essential oils of eucalyptus, cypress, lavender, and ylang-ylang. Referred to as phytoncides (*phyton* meaning "plant" and *cide* meaning "to kill") by forest bathing researchers, these volatile oils are chemicals smells with myriad uses, both for the trees and for us.

Trees use volatile oils for just about everything. They are essential for both communication and defense. Trees use scent signals to warn their neighbors about an impending insect attack. The smells they release can invite friendly animals to come eat any predatory insects that might be munching away on their leaves or trying to burrow a home in their trunks. They can also act as growth regulators, be used to attract pollinators, and protect trees from microbial infections.

The same scents that trees use for protection against predators are the scents identified as immune boosting and stress dissolving in humans. An experiment that released the smell of Hinoki cypress wood oil into hotel rooms over the course of four days showed increases in natural killer cell activity consistent with forest bathing immune function improvements. A similar experiment in olfactory forest simulation tested relaxation responses after a ninety-second burst of Hinoki cypress leaf oil in an otherwise climate-controlled room. A second group went into a matching room with no smell. The leaf oil stimulated parasympathetic nervous system activity and relaxation, even after just a minute and a half. The same responses are found when comparing no smell with the aroma of rose flower, orange peel, and perilla essential oils.

If the aerosols of the forest have healing power on the immune system and the nervous system, it stands to reason that they have similar effects on other bodily systems as well. Indeed, cypress and cedar wood oil inhalation can lower blood pressure after just one minute. Similarly, α-pinene and limonene, two of the volatile oils found in most conifers, decrease blood pressure after less than two minutes. So, too, does the essential oil of the Taiwan cypress (*Chamaecyparis taiwanensis*). They also have anti-tumor properties, increasing levels of anti-tumor proteins such as perforin, granulysin, and granzymes A/B inside human cells. In addition, γ-terpinene, found in eucalyptus trees and other plants, as well as α-pinene and limonene, all decrease inflammation. Pine oil–infused rooms in a work setting can decrease heart rate and increase wakefulness.

None of these results are surprising to naturopathic doctors, herbalists, *curanderos*, and traditional healers across the world who have worked with plants for generations. Practices of using purified volatile oils as medicine date back to ancient Egypt. The volatile oils in citrus and cypress trees have long been used to calm the nerves and help clear congestion in the upper respiratory tract. Other volatile oils such as citronella and lemon eucalyptus have a long history of use as insect repellents. Anyone who has ever used a camphor-menthol-eucalyptus chest rub for a cough has already witnessed the benefits of aromatic medicine. Fir oil stimulates circulation, can help relieve muscle fatigue, and also works as a decongestant. Other volatile oils are well-known for their antimicrobial properties, such as the essential oil made from the tea tree, *Melaleuca alternifolia*.

Forest bathing is literally bathing in the aromatic medicine of the trees and other plants. The mix is akin to using a diffuser in a large room with the essential oils of many different trees at once, plus all the other benefits of being outside. You might think that more is better, but not in the case of volatile oils. Exposure to weak concentrations of α-pinene described as a "slight odor" results in relaxation and decreased stress; exposure to high concentrations and a "strong smell," on the other hand, leads to an increased stress state that people describe as uncomfortable. Dose matters, and the forest delivers just the right amount.

TREE MEDICINE

> I think of the trees and how simply they let go, let fall the riches of a season, how without grief (it seems) they can let go and go deep into their roots for renewal and sleep. . . . Imitate the trees. Learn to lose in order to recover, and remember that nothing stays the same for long, not even pain, psychic pain. Sit it out. Let it all pass. Let it go.
>
> —*May Sarton*

Trees are wise. There is so much you can learn from trees. Many trees are like your grandma, but even older and with more life experience. A few years ago, I had the privilege to hang out with the Great Basin bristlecone pines (*Pinus longaeva*) in the White Mountains of California/Nevada. There, high above the valley, stand the oldest living nonclonal trees in the world. The oldest bristlecone pine is more than 5,000 years old. The second oldest, named Methuselah, is 4,850 years old. Bristlecone pines are a true sight to behold. They have a strikingly different appearance from that of their pine tree cousins at lower altitudes. Bristlecone pines are short and stalky, with gnarled, spiraling trunks and branches that look like the rocks sculpted by centuries of wind erosion in the Altiplano region of Bolivia. They often have needles growing only on one side, or even on a single branch, the rest of the tree barren of life but still very much living. These trees look as though they have weathered thousands of years of severe exposure, because they have. They form open stands of forest, with lots of space between them. If you were going to live for thousands of years, you'd probably want a little extra space between you and your neighbor too.

Walking among these trees is like traveling back in time. Some of these trees have stood since 3000 BC, germinating at the end of the Neolithic period and the birth of the Bronze Age. They were born around the same time as Stonehenge was being built, when the pottery wheel was invented in China, and when the Norte Chico civilization emerged in South America. The bristlecone pines have been alive since the time of Egyptian pharaohs and Sumerian cities in Mesopotamia and the Harappan period in the Indus Valley. Early petroglyphs made by Indigenous Australians date back to the same period. The first incarnation of the city of Troy was founded around this time, long before the ancient Greeks made Troy famous as the setting of the Trojan War. It's truly incredible to realize that a tree you are looking at may be older than the Great Pyramid of Giza in Egypt. Some of the bristlecone pines in the Great Basin have stood, unwavering, living peacefully among the Paiute people for thousands of years before the European colonization of North America.

Standing there, you can't help considering the accumulated wisdom and experience of these trees, having outlasted many human settlements and civilizations, as they stand strong but silent atop the mountains. What kinds of stories must these trees have collected? How many human lifetimes have they witnessed? I stood there, as still as the trees, in awe of their fortitude in the face of high-altitude winds and snow. If they could speak, I wondered, what would they say? What advice might they give us to help us withstand our individual and societal stressors?

It's no wonder that many medicinal plants from the high

altitudes of Siberia and other similar environments have been traditionally used for increasing human resilience to stress. Plants such as rhodiola and Siberian ginseng have been studied for their abilities to modulate stress caused by environmental, physical, and even mental-emotional factors. They have been used for increasing energy, enhancing athletic performance, and even alleviating depression. Looking back to the bristlecone pines, I understood why they have served as a symbol of longevity, strength, and perseverance. The bristlecone pines are uniquely able to withstand harsh conditions because of their dense, resinous bark, which helps them resist the changes in weather and protects them from infection and insect invasions. After the long, winding drive and the hike up into the bristlecone pine forest, a forest bathing trip there can help us connect to our strength and resilience by reminding us of own toughness, even if we live a small fraction of the time these trees survive. They can inspire us to stand tall in our uniquely gnarled or imperfect appearance and face the stresses of life with the wisdom of a thousand years.

Trees have long represented this ability to stand strong and tall. We often talk about trees based on their height, none more so than the great coastal redwood (*Sequoia sempervirens*) trees in California, the tallest trees in the world. Towering over everything at 350 feet (107 meters) tall, these redwoods tend to grow straight into the sky, with very few branches to help them balance. Redwoods remind me of the yogic Tree Pose (Vrikshasana), where you stand on one leg, the sole of your other foot pressed against your standing thigh or calf and your arms stretched above your head. This pose, or asana, helps to improve balance and stability. You can't help but concentrate on maintaining a tall posture, just like a coastal redwood.

VITAMINS G & N

Time spent amongst [sic] trees is never wasted time.

—*Katrina Mayer*

The standardized extract or active constituent of time spent in nature is elusive. It is almost impossible to parse out all the factors involved in the health benefits derived from the interplay between person and environment. Although much of the Japanese research has focused on the role of volatile oils released by trees, the benefits of forest bathing can't be pinned down to just one way of working. Trees help us clean up our air. They remove pollution, especially in our cities. Better air quality leads to better health outcomes, especially in terms of conditions such as asthma.

Expertise and research from other fields point to other factors. Environmental psychologists have shown that green spaces reduce stress while increasing feelings of safety, social integration, and other healthy lifestyle behaviors, including exercise. Children's health researchers have shown that sensory stimulation, visual focus, and field of view are also salient factors, in particular in the research regarding children and ADHD. Increased exposure to sunlight and vitamin D as people spend more time outside is also likely involved.

Conifer trees may expose us to phytoncides, but forests also expose us to the bacteria that make up the forest microbiome, the trees' mix of probiotics. Some experts suggest that being in forests helps to reset and rebalance our own microbiomes. Drawing from theories about the hygiene hypothesis, naturopathic doctor Alan Logan has theorized that gray spaces in our urban centers promote dysbiosis, while green and blue spaces relate to healthier microbiomes. The research hasn't been done yet, but it's possible that forest bathing, through exposure to healthy bacteria, can work to shift our gut flora in similar ways to probiotics and in gentler, more subtle ways than a fecal transplant.

Considering all these factors, how forest bathing works keeps leading us back under the umbrella of the *vis medicatrix naturae*, the healing power of nature. Forest bathing works because nature is healing. Besides, we could all use more vitamin G for green and N for nature.

3

HOW TO FOREST BATHE

Forest bathing is simple. Absolutely anyone can do it, whether young or old, able-bodied or living with a disability. You don't need to be super fit or flexible. It doesn't matter what kind of body you have.

You just need a forest and you. Maybe you don't have easy access to a forest. A park with a lot of trees will do. Don't have a park, a single tree will do. Don't have a tree, a picture of a forest will do.

There is absolutely no wrong way to forest bathe. Go into a forest or sit under a tree. Let five, ten, thirty minutes or more pass, and *bam!* You just forest bathed. Go for a walk through a city park—that's forest bathing too. Unless you've been living under a rock, you've already practiced forest bathing many times without knowing it.

Forest bathing is also quite accessible. Maybe you don't have a forest in your backyard or a car to drive out to a nature reserve. That's okay. Thankfully, many cities have set aside space for parks and have actively planted trees. One of the best things about forest bathing is that it doesn't have to be perfect and there really is no wrong way to do it.

Forest bathing is inexpensive. You don't need any special gear. All you need are trees. Any kind of comfortable clothing works, whatever comfortable means to you. Although you might find it challenging to walk in high heels on the forest floor, there's nothing stopping you from doing it. The most important rule about forest bathing is that you should be yourself. Forest bathing is about finding your own connection (or reconnection) to nature. You can follow some of the exercises I use and write about here, or you can invent your own. You can venture out and make up the rules as you go, or you can join a guided forest bathing group. And you can wear your heels if you want to.

All that said, you might want to dress for the weather. Nothing spoils a forest bathing experience more than getting too cold or too hot or getting a sunburn (yes, the tree leaves will filter out some of the sun's rays and provide shade, but you can still get a sunburn). You might not feel so relaxed if you get rained on without an umbrella or a rain jacket. There is no such thing as bad weather, only inappropriate clothing. Don't let harsh conditions stop you from being outside, but as the Scouts say, be prepared.

Two of my least favorite forest bathing experiences ever involved biting insects. Once, I was lying in our family tent in the Florida Keys in the dark when I realized that the mesh netting seemed to be letting in the no-see-ums. There was not much to do at that point except hide inside my sleeping bag and wait until morning to see how bad the bites were. The other time was a hiking trip I planned for my fortieth birthday. Even though it had snowed just days before, it was May and you couldn't stop walking or you'd be swarmed by blackflies within five seconds. Learn from my mistakes. Bring along your bug spray, check your local weather, pack plenty of water and extra layers of clothing, and get outside.

Don't let your assumptions about what you should do take over from what you want to do or what you are curious about. Allow your natural curiosity to guide your experience while forest bathing. Look at the forest as though you are seeing it through the eyes of a child. Imagine you are seeing and smelling and touching everything for the very first time. Open yourself up to the world as though it is brand-new to you. Allow yourself to be drawn into your forest bathing practice. If you feel called to a specific tree or plant, move toward it and explore it with all of your senses.

Familiarize yourself with the forest as deeply as possible. Become friends with a new tree. Introduce yourself and get the lowdown on your new acquaintance. How does it like to grow? Does it reach straight for the sky or does it wind and curve its way toward the light? How much sunlight does it get? How big is its crown? How do its branches and leaves/needles move with the breeze? What kinds of plants grow at its feet? What animals or insects live harmoniously with this tree? Can you see any of the tree's roots? Learn as much as you can about this single tree sitting in front of you. Get up to speed by slowing down and having fun.

Forest bathing is a practice and a form of play. Become

absorbed in the forest by using your imagination. Look at every rock, tree, and plant as though it has a unique identity and its own history that you can get to know. You need not work toward becoming an expert naturalist. Put down your identification guidebook or your map or your phone and get to know the forest like a new friend. Education or mastery is not the point. The goals of forest bathing are presence, awareness, and relationship, not knowledge and expertise. You might learn about yourself and the forest in the process, but ultimately, forest bathing is about connection.

ACKNOWLEDGMENTS AND GRATITUDE

The first step in forest bathing is to acknowledge the land and its history. Wherever you stand, you were not the first person to do so. In North America, it is more than likely that you or your ancestors were immigrants to this land, as am I. It is with gratitude and an acknowledgment of the history of Indigenous peoples in North America that we are able to stand here, in any forest, today. In other parts of the world, there are likely other people to acknowledge, even if they are your own ancestors.

In any of the walks or forest talks I lead, as well as in my own practice, I start first with expressing gratitude for the care and preservation of the land by the people who came before me. Regardless of your connection to nature or to the Indigenous peoples in the area where you live, you can adapt this gratitude and acknowledgment statement to your local situation and individual values. Here is an example of my statement of acknowledgment and gratitude.

"I'd like to start my forest bathing practice with an acknowledgment that I am here on the Treaty Lands and Territory of the

Mississaugas of the Credit. Long before my family fled persecution in Europe and settled here, this land was also home to the Huron-Wendat and Haudenosaunee. It was part of the Dish with One Spoon Wampum Belt Covenant, an agreement between the Haudenosaunee, Anishinaabe, and allied nations to peaceably share and care for the lands and resources around the Great Lakes. I am grateful for the care and respectful relationships that the people who came before me fostered and nurtured with the trees, animals, plants, and rocks so that I may benefit from them today. Today, the meeting place of T'karonto is still the home to many Indigenous people from across Turtle Island [what we call North America].

"I am grateful to have the opportunity to practice forest bathing in this community, on this land. I commit to treading lightly on the land and making a gentle impact on the environment. I strive to ensure that this land continues to be cared for and treated with respect, for the benefit of generations of plants, animals, and people to come."

MAKE IT EASY

There is no wrong time to forest bathe. You can forest bathe in the morning or after work or whenever you have time. Forest bathing doesn't need to be difficult, like an ascetic exercise of sugar avoidance. It isn't intended to be exhilarating or exhausting like training for a half marathon. It isn't about overcoming the hardship of sitting in silent meditation for hours on end. All of those things might have a positive impact on your health and overall life, but few people would describe them as easy.

Forest bathing doesn't need to be hard, but it is great after a hard day. One of my favorite times to forest bathe is after a long bicycle ride or a stressful day at work. Forest bathing after a period of physical or mental-emotional stress is like shifting the gears of your nervous system to slow down. It's like washing away the grime that's accumulated and basking in sunshine and tree essence.

There's an off-the-grid hostel in Banff National Park that has a wood-burning sauna next to the sleeping cabins that is ideal for forest bathing. After a strenuous hike in the Rocky Mountains to get a glimpse of an ice field or a massive waterfall, it feels like heaven to come home to your hostel in the forest and infuse your tired muscles with a forest bathing session and a dry, hot sauna. You can even run out of the sauna and jump into the cold, natural soaking pool in the creek just outside, all the while surrounded by the giant evergreen trees in the valley below the Rocky Mountain range giants.

Forest bathing doesn't have to be fancy or organized or take a lot of time. You don't even really need any instructions on how to do it. Sit on the grass, lie on a blanket, lean against a tree. If you're feeling ambitious, set up a hammock and then sink into the forest. Bring a friend, bring a snack, bring a book, or bring nothing. If there's anything that has become more clear through research, it's that there is no single correct way to get the health benefits of forest bathing. Every week, a new research study gets published showing that some other aspect of nature is good for your health. So don't stress about the details or doing it right. Just being in a forest is good for you.

It turns out that being around water is pretty great too. Research hasn't yet studied whether being around a forest and a water source is better than either one of them alone, so for now, pick the place that you have the best connection to and go for it. If you're a water person, prioritize sitting in the shade by the coast. If you're a forest person, choose to spend your time on a trail in the mountains next to a glacial spring. The research is clear on one thing: being in nature is good for you.

Forest bathing can be as simple as taking five steps. Take five steps forward into the forest and under the trees. Then use your five senses to guide you in your connection with the forest.

Five senses forest bathing

Five senses forest bathing is an adaptation of a common relaxation exercise that uses the five senses to bring awareness and attention into the present time and space. It is based on a mindfulness exercise that helps you stop feelings of anxiety and panic in their tracks and refocus on the here and now. Using the five senses helps to ground you in the natural environment and to connect you to both the forest and yourself in an active form of meditation.

You can just stand in the forest and get benefits out of the experience, but you might as well do something. Boost your forest bathing practice by drawing on all of your senses. Tactile and olfactory stimulation are critical parts of the forest bathing experience. Touching natural objects such as leaves and tree bark fosters greater relaxation and a deeper sense of calm than touching metal and synthetic fabrics. Research studies confirm what you already know based on personal experience: silk is nicer to the touch than polyester, and wood is warmer and more comforting than steel. It is also clear that scents are paramount to the forest bathing experience. The volatile oils from trees, plants, and flowers can improve immunity, decrease heart rate, and pacify stress hormones, among other things. Passive forest bathing is great for your health.

Active, intentional sensory experiences are only going to amplify these baseline health-promoting effects and make forest bathing truly transformative.

EXERCISE: FIVE SENSES

Look

See the trees, the plants growing underfoot, the fungi, moss, and lichen. Look up, down, and all around for animals hiding under rocks, in burrows, and on tree branches. Bring awareness to the smoothness or roughness of the textures of tree trunk bark. Notice the colors, shapes, and textures of leaves and roots and branches. Count how many different shades of green you can see. Detect the grayish tones of some leaves and the deep forest green of others. Pay attention to the shapes of the leaves, looking out for how thin or thick the needles of conifers grow. Spot the variations in the serration or undulation of leaf margins. Take note of the patterns of venation on the leaves themselves. Consider the tiniest of hairs on the undersides of some leaves.

Look for the patterns in nature, the repetitive shapes or designs. Count the needles on pine trees, the petals of flowers, and the whorled leaves on plants. Satisfy your inner geometry geek and see if you can find the fractals in the world around you. Try to see natural manifestations of the golden ratio or logarithmic spirals in echinacea flowers, pinecones, shells, and riverbeds. Remark on the growth directions and patterns of trees, the specifics of the way the branches emerge from the central trunk. Discern the way the sunlight filters through the trees.

Listen

Listen to the symphony of nature. What does the forest sound like? If you stay still for a few minutes, what can you hear? Yes, if a tree falls in the forest, it does make a sound. A rather loud one, in fact. Different trees make different sounds. Each forest is its own symphony, waiting for you to listen in.

Bask for a moment in your own silence. Plug in to the natural auditory landscape around you. Hear the rustling of leaves, the birdsong, or the running stream water. Listen for the subtle sounds of the forest. Pay attention to the sounds of the little critters scurrying across the forest floor, the slithering of snakes, and the creaking of the tree branches as they sway almost imperceptibly to and fro. Listen to the whispering of the wind and the buzzing of insects. Can you hear a frog croak? Or a wolf or a monkey howl? Can you hear a woodpecker tap, tap, drumming on a tree trunk nearby? What is it trying to say?

Notice the sound of the forest floor under your feet as you shift your weight back and forth or take a single step. Listen for the crinkling of deciduous leaves under your feet or the icy crunching sound of snow. In a coniferous forest, sounds are muffled by the soft layer of dried needles on the forest floor. No matter what kind of forest you are in, if you are quiet enough, you might be able to hear the fizzle-like sound of leaf litter as it settles and decomposes with the help of worms and other bugs.

These are the calmer sounds of the forest, but the forest can also be loud and demonstrate the destructive or transformative power of nature. During a heavy rainfall or a monsoon or an ice storm or a coastal storm surge, the forest can show its full power with the thunderous breaking of massive tree branches or the sound of an entire tree being uprooted and then crashing into its neighbors as it tumbles down. Yes, you will hear that tree fall in the forest—hopefully from a safe distance away.

Smell

Smell the fresh air and the evergreens. As you walk around, smell a few different trees and notice the subtle differences in the scents of different trees. Pay attention to the combinations of volatile oils. Rub an evergreen leaf and take a deep breath. Can you smell the pinene, limonene, camphene, or thujone volatile oils that make up each tree's scent?

Smell the grass and the soil. Squat down and get close to smell a flower as though you are a bee. Try to notice the imperceptible sweetness of a clover flower. Bask in the perfume of lilac flowers or linden or honeysuckle flowers. Smell the combination of scents in the air as the wind blows. Get swept away by the pheromones of the forest.

Feel

Stand or sit still, exactly where you are. Take a moment to feel the ground beneath your feet. Pause a moment to consider your body and its gravity exerting a gentle pressure against the earth. Imagine the same force coming up beneath you, the soil pushing up to meet your feet. Shift your weight back and forth from one foot to the other. Lift one foot at a time and notice if the soil is soft or cushioned or compacted underfoot.

Touch a tree close to you. Notice the texture and strength of the tree trunk. Feel the pattern of the bark across your fingers. Hug a tree. Redefine the term "tree hugger." Feel the softness of the leaves or the grass growing on the ground. Notice if one side of the leaf is different from the other. Feel the prickles of the pinecones and the tickles of the grass. Sink your fingers into a thick, luscious green cushion of moss and watch it bounce back, pushing back against your weight.

If you feel comfortable, take off your shoes. Wiggle your toes on the grass and let the blades gently tickle your feet. Press your heels into the dirt. Get dirty! Imagine yourself connecting to the fungal network underneath your feet. Introduce yourself through the soles of your feet, and watch as your presence percolates and travels through the wood wide web. Spread out your toes and ground yourself into the earth's magnetism. Connect with the forest—skin to skin.

Be cautious if you live near hazardous or toxic plants. When in doubt, stick to the trail and don't touch anything unless you are certain it won't harm you. I have watched unsuspecting trail walkers bend down to touch a leaf of stinging nettle and feel the wrath of its painfully allergic skin response. Last week as I was hiking, I listened to a fellow hiker tell his group that poison ivy can't affect you as long as the leaves are intact. While he's correct that the rash-causing oil is found inside the plant, undamaged plants are incredibly rare, in particular those growing alongside a footpath.

Taste

Taste is the last of the five senses to engage in forest bathing and it's completely optional. Open your mouth to taste the air as it passes or as a drop of rain falls onto your tongue. Try pine-needle or gingko-leaf tea if you have the opportunity. Eat a few lemon-heart leaves if you appreciate tartness. Search for a wild blueberry if the bears haven't gotten to them first. Find the bitter, sweet, sour, salty, pungent, and astringent flavors present in nature and bring them in, to stimulate your digestive and immune systems.

Before you taste anything, it's critical to be 100 percent certain of the identification of the species of tree or plant. Inaccuracy of identification can be the difference between wild carrot and poison hemlock—the former is a survival food and the latter is the poison that famously killed Socrates. Bring a plant expert or a guide or learn about plant identification yourself.

On a recent hike in the Niagara Escarpment, my oldest son challenged me to a one-on-one battle he called "the burdock challenge." The game is played like a staring contest, but with a twist. You both have to eat a palm-sized section of a burdock leaf while keeping a neutral face. The first to flinch loses the game. Burdock leaf is both incredibly fuzzy and unbelievably bitter. Also, I've never been good at poker. I notoriously wear my emotions on my face, and this time was no different. I managed to hold it together for a solid ten chews before I couldn't hold it in any longer. I grimaced. And then I lost. I doubt I'll ever be able to win this challenge, but there really is nothing like a fuzzy, bitter leaf in your mouth to help you focus on the present moment and nothing else. It's mindfulness on steroids.

GO DEEPER

Want to take your forest bathing practice to the next level? Maybe you've been forest bathing for a while, or perhaps your whole life. You love the time you spend in nature and you want to get even more out of the time you have outside. Yes, forest bathing can be simple, and it doesn't need to take a lot of time. Next-level forest bathing is still simple—it's simply the addition or incorporation of another healthy habit or therapy into your practice. This section draws from my naturopathic expertise in herbal medicine, mind-body medicine, and hydrotherapy to show you how to maximize your forest bathing practice and go beyond to seize even greater health benefits.

Tap into tree medicine

Most of the research on forest bathing has been done in a handful of forests in Japan very close to Tokyo, with the same few species of trees. Of course, we know that each forest is unique and has different species of trees and plants. You could perhaps assume that forest bathing works only in those particular Japanese forests with those particular coniferous trees. And you'd be wrong. Research into the health of people living close to green spaces has been conducted primarily in Europe and North America, places with completely different species of trees and wildly different forests. In some ways, the types of trees don't matter. In other ways, they do.

Trees are literally medicine. Many of our routinely used pharmaceuticals have their origins in trees. Pharmaceuticals for all different kinds of acute and chronic illnesses have natural derivatives in trees and plants. Camphor, found in many topical pain relief formulas and inhaled nasal decongestant products, is abundant in the camphor tree native to East Asia and invasive in Australia and the United States, where it has been introduced. Aescin, derived from horse chestnut trees, has been used topically and internally for hemorrhoids. Trees in the *Cinchona* genus from the Andean region of South America were traditionally used to bring down fevers by the Quechua people. Quinine, a chemical found in those trees, has since been manufactured for use as a drug to treat malaria. Paclitaxel, the most well-known natural-source cancer drug, frequently used in the treatment of breast, lung, ovarian, and pancreatic cancers, was originally derived from Pacific yew trees. Even some asthma medications have their roots in trees. Theophylline, a drug used to dilate the airways in chronic respiratory conditions, comes from the cacao tree, which is much more famous for supplying us with another drug-like substance, chocolate. Probably the most common drug that has its origins in trees is acetylsalicylic acid, more commonly known as aspirin. Acetylsalicylic acid is now produced synthetically but is also found naturally as salicylic acid in willow bark. The salicylic acid in willow acts like the synthetic drug as both a pain reliever and an anti-inflammatory, but without the unfortunate side effect of causing stomach ulcers.

Medicine is hidden deep within the trees, but it is also everywhere around them. That inner medicine permeates the whole tree and even the area around it. It floats in the air in the form of volatile oils but also through the soil and its fungal networks. Sitting in a conifer forest feels different from sitting in a deciduous one. And both of those are completely different from a rain forest or a cloud forest. Every forest has a feeling, an energy that you become a part of as soon as you enter it. Maybe you've noticed something different too.

In my naturopathic medical practice, I often use herbal medicine and combine it with forest bathing. With a deep understanding of the medicinal use and energetics of different trees, I can recommend that patients practice forest bathing next to or underneath the trees that hold the healing qualities they need at that moment in their lives. If I've recommended forest bathing for a patient struggling with depression, I might suggest that they sit under a mimosa tree (*Albizia julibrissin*), whose Chinese name transliterates to "collectively happy." In traditional Chinese herbal medicine, mimosa tree bark and flowers are used to calm the spirit and bring joy back into the heart by relieving constrained emotions such as depression, irritability, and anger. Likewise, if I'm recommending forest bathing for a patient with heart health issues, I might suggest they sit near a hawthorn (*Crataegus sp.*) tree, which has been shown in human clinical research trials to improve symptoms of heart disease and decrease blood pressure.

There's a tree for everyone and every problem. Many years ago, I had a patient in his late twenties come to my office with chronic back pain. His back pain had started when his father had passed away and he was tasked with renovating his family home to get it ready to sell. He was bent over, sanding and then refinishing the house's wood floors, when the pain first started to set in. Months later, he still found it painful to sit at his desk and work on his computer for long periods of time. By the end of the day, he didn't have it in him to go out or play baseball with his friends because the pain was exhausting. He was taking the daily maximum dose of over-the-counter painkillers, but he was worried about the long-term effects on his stomach and liver. When I asked him to describe the pain, he said his lower back felt like a stiff plank of wood. He was also feeling pessimistic about his recovery and his life after losing his dad when he was so young.

In addition to gentle stretches and recovery exercises, I recommended he switch to willow bark for pain relief. Ancient Egyptians and Native North Americans used willow bark for alleviating pain and fever, as did Hippocrates, who wrote about it in the fifth century BC. Research on willow bark for people with osteoarthritis shows that it works as advertised.

Taking willow bark for his pain was good, but taking willow bark for his pain and sitting under a willow tree was even better. My children used to call willows "monkey trees" because they always hoped to see a monkey swinging from one branch to the next. Whenever they get the chance, they too would swing from a willow's branches. Willow branches are known for their flexibility. They are thin but strong and bend easily. Weeping willow branches seem to be constantly moving downward, like a rain shower of narrow gray-green leaves or like the slow, glittering trail of fireworks as they fizzle out.

Historically, willow branches were used to make rounded structures, skirts and baskets, because they bend easily and can be formed into arches or woven into fabrics. In Taoism, willow represents the concept of strength in weakness. Willow bark helped this patient increase his emotional pliability and adaptability without losing the sense of his grief. It helped him to move more freely and without pain and increased his sense of optimism. After a couple of weeks of forest bathing with a willow tree at his local park, he noted that both his back and his thoughts felt less rigid.

Trees have loads of medicine to offer if you take the time to get to know them. Aside from the benefits of essential oils and specific medicinal qualities, trees in their most basic function are our complementary living beings. We have a special relationship with trees. Humans and trees are deeply interconnected.

Humans rely on oxygen in the air to survive. With each breath, we draw oxygen into our lungs. In the tiniest parts of our lungs, the alveoli, that oxygen is exchanged with carbon dioxide. We then breathe out the carbon dioxide and, without even thinking about it, breathe in oxygen once again. We repeat this process, breathing in and out, exchanging oxygen for carbon dioxide, more than twenty thousand times a day. We use oxygen in almost every biochemical reaction in our bodies. It fuels our energy production and our absorption and our cellular regeneration.

Trees, our natural partners in breath, do exactly the opposite. During photosynthesis, trees convert energy from sunlight to make glucose from carbon dioxide and water. Oxygen is merely a by-product of this process. Trees do use some of this oxygen for energy production, but there is a net excess, which gets released in the environment. How much oxygen a single tree produces depends on the species, its age, its health, and its surroundings. Estimates suggest that one tree can produce anywhere from 220 to 265 pounds (100 to 120 kilograms) of oxygen per year. Humans, on the other hand, breathe in approximately 1,650 to 1,985 pounds (750 to 900 kilograms) of oxygen per year. Although that number can vary greatly depending on exercise and the air's concentration of oxygen, which decreases at higher altitudes, we need about seven or eight trees to support the oxygen intake of one human per year. Of the oxygen that we breathe in, we use about 5 percent of it and breathe the rest out, along with carbon dioxide.

In an oversimplified sense, trees breathe in carbon dioxide and breathe out oxygen. We literally breathe in what trees breathe out. This process is important in terms of preserving our environment, especially in preventing climate change and protecting the ozone layer. However, it is also critical in ensuring we have enough energy to get through our days.

As you forest bathe, you can activate this special relationship with trees just by breathing. You don't need to change your breath in any way or count your inhalations and exhalations. Tree breathing is an easy way to initiate a relationship and connection with forests and nature.

EXERCISE: TREE BREATHING

Use this simple breathing exercise to amplify your forest bathing experience. Start by finding a tree. Choose any tree you are interested in or curious about or find visually appealing. Sit or stand facing the tree. Find a comfortable position and start to breathe. You need not change your breath in any way. It doesn't matter if your breath is slow or fast, deep or shallow. Just breathe in and out. Feel free to close your eyes if you want. If you do, you can picture your breath moving in and out of your body in your mind.

Continue breathing in and out. With each inhalation, or breath in, visualize or imagine the oxygen coming from the tree in through your nose or mouth and traveling down into your lungs. Pause for a second to imagine a trade-off—oxygen goes into your bloodstream and carbon dioxide comes out. As you exhale, or breathe out, visualize the carbon dioxide leaving your body and the tree opposite you taking it in through its leaves. With your next inhale, imagine that the oxygen the tree has thrown out as waste is the same oxygen you breathe in. Continue the visualization, breathing in and out in rhythm with the tree.

EXERCISE: STAND TALL

This forest bathing exercise can help you to adopt the fortitude, perseverance, and resilience of trees. Trees face innumerable obstacles throughout their long lives, yet they continue to reach for the sun. Like the yoga asana Vrikshasana, or Tree Pose, this exercise is grounding and helps with balance, concentration, and stability in both mind and body. It can also help you to center yourself in your values and beliefs and find strength in your unique authenticity.

Look around for a tall tree that embodies a growth pattern you admire or find inspiring. The tree can be a straight conifer or a spiny honey locust or a gnarly juniper. Stand near or in view of this tree. Begin by planting both feet firmly on the ground. Feel each corner of your foot and each one of your toes pressing down into the ground, and sense the ground pushing back up against your feet. Evenly distribute your weight between both feet. Take a deep breath in and draw the security and strength of the earth up through the soles of your feet into your torso and continuing up through your head. As you exhale, concentrate that sense of connection and groundedness into your core. Inhale again, deriving power once more from the ground into your body and conserving it in your center. Continue breathing in and out, building upon this feeling of groundedness. In your mind's eye, visualize roots extending down from the soles of your feet and out from the tips of your toes, spreading to secure you to this spot where you stand. Stand tall and firm in this space.

If you are comfortable, you can continue this exercise while adopting the stance of the tree you have chosen. For example, if you choose a tall, straight pine tree, you might raise your arms overhead and reach for the sky. If you admire the beauty of a twisty tree, allow your body to curve and twist in a way that feels good to you. If you appreciate the thorniness of some trees, imagine growing spikes of your own. Regardless of the kind of tree pose you adopt, be sure to keep your feet planted firmly on the ground. Breathe with your tree for another moment or two, harmonizing yourself with your tree. When you are ready, focus your breath back into your chest or belly, release your connection with the ground, and slowly take a step.

Practice mindfulness outdoors

The five senses forest bathing exercise is essentially one form of mindfulness. Mindfulness is merely the practice of bringing awareness to the inner workings of the mind and body. Many of my patients mistakenly believe that the goal of mindfulness or meditation is to empty your mind of thought and think about nothing at all. What a lofty goal that would be! They frequently express resistance to the idea of mindfulness because they think about mindfulness only as practiced in the silent style of Buddhist meditation. Mindfulness, however, can be considered as a general concept. Any time you are bringing awareness to your mind, you are being mindful. Mindfulness is practicing being aware of the present moment that you find yourself in, while calmly acknowledging, naming, and accepting your bodily sensations, feelings, or thoughts.

Mindfulness is a great companion to forest bathing, especially for those people who struggle with sitting forms of meditation. I've never been proficient at the standard silent meditation or the kinds of meditation where you focus on the breath, mostly while sitting down. I realized that my most mindful moments were likely to come not when I was sitting still but rather when I was moving around. I was calmest and most peaceful and most grateful when I was randomly but rhythmically walking or dancing or doing something repetitive like knitting or pulling weeds out of the garden. Forest bathing is the ideal meditative practice for people who like to move.

Gratitude practice is another style of mindfulness that

seamlessly incorporates into forest bathing. Appreciation of the one thing right there and then. Appreciate the macroscopic things, like the tiny patterns on the wings of butterflies or the finely toothed leaf edges of a black cherry tree or a red maple. Treasure the big things, the majesty of the tallest trees, the fluffiness of clouds, the warmth of the sun, the vastness of the sky. At dusk, admire the colors of the sunset. Set foot outside at night and search for the immensity of constellations and the Milky Way. Give thanks for the time you are taking for yourself and the intention you are setting to relax and cope with life's stressors in a positive way. Say thank you to the forest. Say thank you to yourself.

EXERCISE: SIT SPOT

A sit spot is a place of quiet awareness. It can be anywhere, but a forest bathing sit spot is always outside. Most people have a spot they are naturally drawn to over and over again. It's the spot where you instinctively want to sit down for a while and contemplate the universe. I have sit spots in different parks all over my city, places that feel restful and calm and rejuvenating. One of my sit spots is at the top of a hill that overlooks the off-leash dog park in the park by my house. In another park, my sit spot is on a large boulder underneath an old oak tree with a view of the river.

Find a sit spot in a park or a forest or your backyard or wherever you are in nature (ideally a place you can easily return to). Some people are drawn to a sit spot that has a wide perspective, while others are drawn to a place that is more like a nest or cove-like space that they can look out from as they might a hiding spot. Look around and let your heart guide you to a place to sit down. If you have trouble sitting, find a place to stand or lean. Get comfortable. Stay quietly in place for one minute or five minutes or thirty minutes. How much time you spend doesn't matter, it's how you spend the time. Focus on observing the natural world around you. You can use the five senses exercise as a guide or just be present in the moment.

The sit spot exercise isn't a onetime deal. It works slowly, over time. Each time you come back to your sit spot, you might notice what is the same and what is different. Visiting your sit spot at different times of the day and in different seasons will help you to get to know your sit spot even better. You might notice which birds sing in the morning and which sing at night. You might have the privilege of familiarizing yourself with the timing of flowers blooming or the way the trees respond to the wind. You might begin to witness patterns and rhythms. Sooner or later, you may perceive a deepening of your relationship to nature and your connection to place. If you want, bring a notebook with you to jot down your observations or your reflections. Over time, many people find that their sit spot becomes a place that anchors them in their life, a place where they can go to cultivate presence, a space that connects them through the present to their past and their future.

EXERCISE: LETTING GO

This exercise is best performed in autumn in temperate forests across North America, when the deciduous trees change color and let go of their leaves in preparation for winter. If you live in subtropical or tropical areas, this exercise is best timed when trees lose their leaves at the beginning of the dry season.

Trees shed their leaves to help them to conserve water and energy. As the weather gets colder, hormones in the trees are released to trigger the tree to reabsorb nutrients from the leaves and then cut them off through a process called "abscission." Leaves change from green to yellow, orange, and red as the chlorophyll, which gives leaves their green color, is broken down.

Holding on to extraneous parts during the cold winter months doesn't make sense to trees. That's why they let go of leaves in the fall and re-create themselves in the spring. Holding on to unnecessary parts of ourselves doesn't make sense either. Fall is a great time for shedding old ideas or bad habits. It is a natural time for letting go of anything that we don't want to hold on to anymore.

Find a sit spot near one or more trees that are losing their leaves. Think about one specific thing that you want to let go of or let be. Maybe it's a negative thought you have been carrying around about yourself. Maybe you want to mark a new stage of your grieving process for a loved one. Maybe you have been struggling to stop a bad habit and are wanting to start the winter off with healthier coping mechanisms. Maybe you want to let go of something painful in your past.

With open or closed eyes, picture whatever you want to let go of and place it into a leaf. If you have what feels like a lot to release, visualize it going into many leaves on the same branch, either together or one by one. Say good-bye to it. See it in the leaf. In your mind's eye, see those leaves losing their connection to the tree branch and falling to the ground. Imagine them being covered with snow. Watch them decompose. Say good-bye again. Repeat this visualization as many times as you want, to assist you in your mindfulness practice of letting go. Feel the space you have opened up in yourself, an airy lightness, the space you can fill with new memories or habits or thoughts. Send compassion and gratitude to yourself and the trees for this exercise and their gentle reminder of the cycles of life.

Fall in love

Forest bathing can inspire you to find beauty in something new or unexpected. When you approach forest bathing as a meditative practice with the curiosity of an awe-filled child, you never know what mysteriously beautiful new-to-you object of affection you might find.

Forest bathing can be like falling in love. In those moments of silence, when you're practicing forest bathing and noticing the world around you, you can transcend the ordinary and find the extraordinary. As you use your eyes as though you've never seen what is in front of you ever before, the trees magically come to life in ways previously unimaginable. Trees can be stylish and stand out from the crowd. Branches can dance to the music of the wind.

During my last trip to Taiwan, I fell in love at first sight. It was lightning speed, even though my electric scooter maxed out at 18.6 miles per hour (30 kilometers per hour). I was on a small island highway crossing several islands in the archipelago of the Taiwan Strait. The sun was blazing hot and I was greasy with layers of sunscreen. I felt compelled to stop and stand in the power, and shade, of this tree I had never seen before.

It was a conifer, to be sure. Like most conifers, it had a straight trunk, shooting upward like a rocket. It was the overall shape of the tree that had caught my eye. The needles were short and covered the branchlets like spruce. They resembled long green fingers reaching up to grab the sky. The tree was almost perfectly symmetrical and pyramidal, with widely separated branches, giving it the appearance of a sparse synthetic Christmas tree, but the most beautiful one you have ever seen. I later learned my new love's name is Norfolk Island pine (*Araucaria heterophylla*), which isn't a pine tree at all but is cultivated and sold as an indoor potted Christmas ornamental.

The real magic was coming home. I drove from Toronto to Ottawa to pick up my children. Watching the trees that line the highway, I rekindled old flames. I was jet-lagged and it was early in the morning. The morning dew was thick as fog. The sun was pressing through the clouds, breaking through with a few short beams of light. The light hit the red bark of the eastern red cedar tree and I immediately knew I was home. My heart filled with a new love for my old favorite tree. My soul refueled, I smiled and kept driving.

It's no wonder we use the word "rekindled" when talking about finding new joys in old loves. To rekindle means to stir up and arouse anew, to burn again the flame that has fizzled out. It has the same origin as the word "kindling," those little pieces of dry wood I get my children to collect when we're camping that you need to start a fire.

As I write this book, I am sitting under a willow tree on a large rock with my laptop. I am grateful to be here, in the shade, beside one of Toronto's rivers, breathing in the smell of grass and spruce trees, listening to the call of the red-winged blackbirds. Just now I heard a thunk beside me. Two seagulls had been fighting over a fish one of them had caught, and it dropped to the ground; the owner swooped low to pick it up and flew back over the water again. There is a deer crossing the river, lapping up the water and carefully traversing to the bank on the other side. I turn my head and there is a monarch butterfly flitting past me. It almost feels like a utopian dream. For a moment, it doesn't feel like the city. Gone are the writing deadlines, the pages of lab work from patients to review, and student evaluations to complete. I smile, drunk on the beauty of it all, and get back to writing.

Forest bathing shares in this potential for renewal. It can reawaken your spirit and rekindle your love of nature. It can stir deep feelings and transform you into a butterfly. Allowing yourself this time outside, in the woods, either alone or with others, can give you the space to find gratitude, self-compassion, and even love. In those moments of quiet reflection and observation of yourself and your surroundings, you open yourself up to great potential. For some, this time can catalyze profound soul healing. Some patients have remarked to me that they forgave themselves some long-forgotten trespass during a forest bathing session or finally let go of some specific line of repetitive negative thinking they had held on to since childhood. Others mention that they find themselves appreciating the present moment enough to bring a sense of calm or joy or even bliss. All of them discern a difference within themselves—an interest or passion or playfulness once asleep, now woken. Let the forest intermingle with your spirit and rekindle an old flame.

EXERCISE: HEART TO HEART

Heart to heart is an exercise that helps you to regulate your own heartbeat while tapping into the heartbeat of a tree. It combines an exercise in listening to trees with a simple technique for increasing coherence between your breath and your emotions. Increasing coherence reduces both the feelings and the physical symptoms associated with stress, which in turn decreases heart rate as well as heart rate variability. Trees don't actually have heartbeats, but they do make sounds as their sap moves up and down their trunks. Using a stethoscope, you can hear the sounds of fluid traveling in some hardwood trees, especially in the spring when the sap is running. Although it can be fun to listen to the gurgling and bubbling sounds from inside a tree, you don't need a stethoscope for this exercise.

Choose a tree to stand beside or sit next to. Place one hand on the trunk of the tree. With closed eyes, use your fingertips to listen to the tree. Can you feel any movement underneath the bark? Can you hear the tree's sap flowing? Imagine the tree transporting vital nutrients up and down the trunk through the sap. Connect to the nourishment that the movement represents. Just as the tree uses its sap to transfer nutrients from roots to leaves, so too does your heart use the flow of blood to nourish all the cells in your body—from roots to leaves and from head to toe.

Place your other hand on your chest over your heart. Focus your attention on this area and imagine your breath flowing in and out of your heart. Sense the smooth movement of blood, oxygen, and other nutrients from your heart out toward your fingers and your toes. Let your breath become a little slower, and a little deeper, as you concentrate on building strength through your heart center. Bring to mind a positive feeling such as appreciation or caring or love for someone or something in your life. Capture this feeling of ease, calmness, and relaxation as you connect to yourself and to the tree.

Get wet with hydrotherapy

Green and blue spaces are rarely separate in nature. Forests can be found alongside streams and rivers and lakes. Even if we can't see the water, it is there—as dew on the leaves in the morning, running in underground trickles to feed the roots of the trees, nourishing the tree trunks and helping to move nutrients between the trees, and feeding the trees on the mountainsides with glacial spring water. Just as forests and trees need water to survive, so do we. The earth's surface is around 70 percent water; our bodies are around 60 percent. Trees, too, have almost as much liquid inside them as we do.

Trees exhale gallons of water a day through a process called "transpiration." You can't see it, but transpiration works like a vacuum, creating a suction that helps the tree draw water upward through its tiny vessels. Water is also drawn upward through osmosis, as water moves from cells with less sugar to cells with more sugar to even out the percentage of water in all the cells. Even still, transpiration and osmosis can't account for all the water inside a tree's trunk. You can't see the water, but sometimes you can actually hear it. In the spring, when water pressure in the trees is at its peak, you can listen in with a stethoscope to the beating heart of the tree. Much of the relationship between forests and water still remains a mystery.

Doctors and medicine people around the world have traditionally understood this integral connection between health and water. European and North American doctors working in the 1800s frequently used hydrotherapy, the therapeutic use of water, alongside other techniques to help move the patient toward health. Hydrotherapy was used in sanatoriums, health retreats, and medicinal spas in between outdoor rest periods and therapeutic exercise. Dew walking was a hydrotherapy technique used by these nature doctors that fits perfectly into a forest bathing practice.

EXERCISE: DEW WALKING

Dew walking is a simple but seemingly magical way to say hello to your morning and walk away feeling refreshed and ready to start your day. Sparkling, early morning dew has fascinated people for centuries. Dew seems like a magical substance. Water droplets almost appear to float like pearls on the surface of leaves, glistening in the warm, orange light of the morning sun. Dew is somehow both fluid and static, like liquid mercury. This resemblance is why it has long been the symbol of transformation and the philosopher's stone, the mystical alchemic substance capable of turning everyday metals into gold. Walking on dewy grass in the morning isn't going to turn you into King Midas, but it can become a revitalizing morning ritual.

Like many hydrotherapy techniques, dew walking works by increasing circulation. The cool dew on your feet triggers temperature receptors that signal to your blood vessels near the surface to quickly constrict to avoid heat loss. A short time later, those same blood vessels relax to help bring warm blood to the skin's surface of your feet. Since cold-water applications on your feet draw blood from the rest of the body to help warm you up, dew walking can help to relieve congestive headaches. Walking helps to magnify these effects. Using your leg muscles helps your blood move against gravity by creating a venous pump. With increased local blood circulation, more nutrients, oxygen, and immune cells can get where they need to go and waste products can be cleared away. Increasing lower leg and foot circulation may help people with varicose veins and those with perpetually cold hands and feet. It can also promote faster wound healing and improve other leg and feet conditions such as diabetic neuropathy and peripheral artery disease.

Going barefoot also has other advantages. It activates receptors on your feet that work on proprioception, the sense of your body in space. Woken up by movement and pressure, proprioceptors tell you where you are, what the terrain is like, and where you are going. The job of these receptors is to make sure you don't whack your toes into the door frame, but they're also used by the brain to make subtle changes in your balance and your gait. Barefoot walking can help to improve balance and proprioception, which is one of the reasons many pediatricians and orthopedic specialists today recommend zero drop or thin-soled shoes for both children and adults.

For your first dew-walking experience, start in the summer. Find a grassy spot that looks welcoming to stand on. Ease your way into winter dew walking by first growing accustomed to more tolerable temperatures under your feet. Before you start, make sure your feet are warm. Run them under warm water if you need to. Head outside to a grassy area and take off those shoes and socks. Walk around the area or walk on the spot for two to three minutes. Take it slow. Savor each step as it approaches the cool wetness of the grass blades in the morning.

If you're brave enough, or an old hand at dew walking, you can wake up your circulation quickly by snow walking. Snow walking is intense, so you should do it for only thirty seconds or so. You're not trying to be like the Iceman, Wim Hof. Or maybe you are. Either way, don't rush. Take it slow and build up your tolerance to extreme temperatures.

Keep a pair of dry socks handy and put on your socks and shoes after you've completed your dew walk. Continue to walk around for another minute to keep the circulation in your legs and feet moving and to warm your feet up again before continuing on with your day.

Make it social

Forest bathing by yourself can be quiet, meditative, and private. It's a gift of solitude and contemplation that Thoreau would be proud of. Solo forest bathing is ideal for introverts or when you just need to escape from the daily grind. Communal forest bathing, on the other hand, satisfies the extrovert in you that wants to share this amazing practice with someone else.

Forest bathing with others offers unique benefits that forest bathing by yourself can't achieve. When you share in an experience with someone or several other people, even if you don't talk about it while it's happening, the feelings are often magnified several times over. Like when you watch a movie with friends and then you review it together after you leave the theater. Forest bathing with friends and family is rewarding in a whole other way.

Group forest bathing helps create a sense of connection among everyone doing it together. It bonds the shared experience and instills feelings of belonging and safety and mutual care. Often you are forced to recognize your interdependence when you are outside forest bathing in a group, as you become aware of how others interact in the space or you look out for poison ivy on the trail. It's a little bit easier to understand someone else's point of view once you've tried to see the image of the cat or the reclining Buddha figure that your friend sees in the clouds. You profoundly grasp the subjectivity of the human experience and reach new heights of empathy. It's no wonder research shows that forest bathing decreases aggression in children and increases cooperation.

Trees are a powerful reminder of our connections. Just as a single tree is connected to other trees in its stand and each stand is connected to other stands in a forest, so too are humans connected to one another in the communities we form. Tree communities can help to create and deepen not only our connections to nature but also our relationships with one another.

EXERCISE: SHARE THE LOVE

Create a community of forest bathers. Invite your friends and family to join you in your forest bathing. Start a regularly scheduled forest bathing meet-up. Grab a colleague and head to the park during lunch. Go to a meeting for the local "friends of" your city park group. Join a forest bathing group. Share your love of forest bathing with others by talking about your forest bathing practice or a specific part of your observations or experience.

Document your forest bathing experience to share with others, both in person and online. Make notes of your reflections, write a poem inspired by the forest, or sketch a picture of a new tree or plant you encountered. Turn your phone back on and take a picture of your forest bathing setting or a selfie of you basking in a forest glow. Share your creations on social media and spread the love of #forestbathing. Connect with other nature lovers in your neighborhood and around the world.

FOREST BATHING AS A WAY OF LIFE

Incorporate nature and forest bathing into your daily life. Don't think about it as an extra thing you need to put on your to-do list. Instead, focus on how you can prescribe more green to yourself without it becoming onerous and a chore. Just as with exercise, you can love it or hate it. You just need to do it, since you know it's good for you. Once forest bathing becomes part of your routine and your daily lifestyle, you won't need to remind yourself to do it. Forest bathing will work, even if you think it's as awful as laundry or washing the dishes. Incorporate it into your life, and it will do the rest. You'll probably grow to love it.

Get off public transit one or more stops early to walk through a park. Cycle or in-line skate to school or work. Eat your lunch outside or go for a walk on a break. If you have trees in your yard, stop for a moment or two before you walk in the door. Surround yourself with green. Grow plants, inside your house or out. If you don't have space for a garden, use pots. Put up pictures of appealing landscapes to look at from time to time. Plant a tree. Swim in a lake. Sit in the park for a picnic. Visit a botanical garden. Wander through a cemetery. Find a nice bench or rock with a good view and just sit.

I'm lucky to have been able to incorporate forest bathing so much into my daily life. I have written this book on a porch or hammock or dock beside a lake, staring out the window at a subtropical forest beside a gorge in Taiwan, and in the sanctity of my backyard in the city under the shade of an overgrown plum tree. How can you shift your life to spend more of it basking in nature?

Workout outside

Get active and do it outside. Green exercise is a two-for-one deal. You get physically active and more fit *and* you receive the benefits of forest bathing. Invite a friend for a hike. Organize a game of softball or football or basketball outside. Help clean up a local park. Go snowshoeing or cross-country skiing. Walk a dog. Get dirty. Start gardening. Do yoga in the park. Do the Tree Pose with actual trees. There are endless ways to incorporate the philosophies of forest bathing and *friluftsliv* into your life.

Being outside is good for your health, even without the benefit of exercise. But if you do choose to exercise in nature, studies show that you'll feel a greater sense of revitalization, energy, enjoyment, and satisfaction. In one study on forest bathing for people with chronic neck pain, forest bathing by itself was compared with forest bathing plus stretching and strengthening rehabilitation exercises. Both groups noted significant decreases in pain, and the study participants were able to move their necks more freely after five two-hour daily sessions of forest bathing. In the group that also did stretching and strengthening, the number of painful trigger points was substantially lower than with those who forest bathed alone.

Walk everywhere

Walking to where you want to go makes it easy to incorporate forest bathing into your life. Maximize your travel time by planning your route based on nature exposure. Map out your route so you can walk through a city park or under a tree canopy. Where possible, have a walking meeting with work colleagues instead of sitting in a stuffy boardroom. Just keep moving. Get off public transit one or two stops early.

When I was in naturopathic medical school, I traveled to and from school by subway. The fastest route had me take one train east and then connect to another train line heading north. The east–west route was notoriously crowded and I always felt a little grumpier after jostling for space inside the sardine-can train car. After a couple of weeks, I grew weary of my morning commute. It's hard to look forward to starting your day getting pushed like a domino every time the train starts or stops. On a whim, one day I decided to walk to the closest station on the north–south train line instead of heading to the station closest to my apartment. I meandered my way through the residential streets and then a park before I reached the station about twenty-five minutes away. Standing on the train platform that morning, I realized how calm and happy I was compared with the usual distaste I had for my commute. It may have added about five or ten minutes to my morning, but the positivity was worth it. Ever since, I have always considered how pleasant a route might be in deciding how to get from here to there.

My own experiences are supported by research on university students walking around campus. Even though university students couldn't predict that walking outside would improve their moods, traveling outside between classes rather than using underground walkways and tunnels resulted in more positive and optimistic mental outlooks. This research confirms that forest bathing and nature exposure don't have to be separated from day-to-day activities, nor do they have to be time-consuming. Even ten to fifteen minutes a day has a profound impact on perception and mood.

Plant a tree or a hundred

Planting trees makes forest bathing that much more accessible for everyone. More trees equals more forest bathing. The greater the tree canopy over our cities, the better. Creating spaces for trees in all the corners of our cities could help reduce social disparities and increase health equity for everyone. Trees have endless health and environmental benefits, but they also have social, cultural, and economic benefits too.

Parks with trees provide a social and community connection. Over the past twenty years, I've watched my local urban park transform into an outdoor community hub. On any summer day, you can see people participating in many different activities. There are people walking their dogs and cycling on the paths. Others might be playing baseball or soccer or throwing a Frisbee. Some people will be sitting in the shade of a large tree having a picnic, meeting up with friends, or going on dates. In between the trees, there are usually people balancing on slack ropes. Another area is perfect for setting up cricket games. Trees are used to mark goalposts and hang balloons from. Children are swinging and sliding on play structures and digging in the sand and climbing trees. Some days, the park looks a little bit like a music festival; other days, there actually is a music festival in the park. On Tuesdays, there is a farmers' market. A few times during the summer, there is an outdoor movie night.

There are lots of other reasons to plant trees to make more forests for bathing in. Trees have other social and economic benefits. Aside from the ones already mentioned, trees provide beauty, increased property values, soil erosion prevention, stormwater reductions, noise reductions, and cultural value.

We plant trees to remember people and mark a place in our hearts. Trees are often partners in our grieving process, a heart-filled symbol of someone or something. As with a gravestone or an altar, people flock to these special trees to pray, to remember, and to pay homage to a person or a piece of history. The tree you planted in remembrance of someone or something is a powerful place to forest bathe.

Planting a tree is the ultimate exercise in optimism. When you plant a sapling, you are planting for the future. A single tree can easily live several hundred years. Planting a tree is like a commitment to the future, a gift to generations to come. It is a vow to believe in the promise of tomorrow, to remain positive in spite of life's ups and downs. Putting a tree into the ground with the knowledge that it will outlive you by hundreds of years demonstrates a recognition of your place in universal time, a responsibility for the people not yet born, and a faithfulness to life itself.

{ 4 }

FAQS

WHAT IF I'M ALLERGIC TO TREES?

Allergic to trees? Bedridden? If you really can't make it out into nature, it's no problem. While you won't necessarily get all the health benefits of forest bathing, there are still plenty of ways to get at least some of the positive benefits of getting outside. The great news is that plenty of research shows that even looking at pictures or videos of nature works.

Patients in hospital rooms that look out over green scenes recover faster from surgery. People who have to undergo painful procedures such as biopsies say they feel less pain if they are looking at a picture of a natural landscape than do people staring at the fluorescent lights on the bare ceiling. One study had people watch a stressful movie and then watch either natural- or urban-setting videos. When they compared the groups, the people who watched videos of natural settings recovered from the stress faster and more completely than the people who saw videos of urban settings. Other research studies show similar results. Looking at nature scenes activates the anterior cingulate cortex and the insula, parts of the brain associated with emotional stability, love, empathy, and altruistic motivation. Looking at urban scenes, on the other hand, activates the amygdala, the part of the brain associated with responses to adverse, dangerous, or fearful situations. Looking at nature shifts our perceptions.

Clinicians and researchers agree that looking at images of nature induces psychological feelings of calmness and relaxation. It also induces physiological relaxation by releasing muscle tension and normalizing heart rates. It encourages greater body positivity and self-image. It doesn't matter what type of landscape the images depict, either. Images and videos from kiwifruit orchards to forested landscapes to seascapes all result in greater relaxation, lower heart rates, and more sustained feelings of wakefulness. All the more so if the person's preferred landscape is the one being looked at. The takeaway here is that you should look at pictures or videos of your preferred natural environment. Whatever type of landscape you love, just look at it.

Looking at images of nature can be relaxing and decrease pain. It's one of the reasons I decorated my office with landscape photography. Even when we're stuck inside, we can sneak in a little imaginary forest bathing by gazing at natural scenery in any art form. Indoor plants also make a big impact. Memory recall, creativity, mood, and academic scores all improve with incorporating live plants into indoor living environments. Green your house or office to brighten your life. Color psychologists and interior designers understand the impacts of green and blue colors in our indoor environments. Green as a color symbolizes nature and represents health, well-being, and tranquility. Green is calming, as is blue, which represents tranquility, serenity, and safety. It's no wonder that many healing spaces use natural shades of green and blue to enlist the healing power of nature indoors.

Several research studies set out to see if there was a difference between looking at pictures or other representations of nature and actually being next to the living plants and trees. Real or fake, researchers wondered, does it make a difference? Unfortunately, the answer seems to be that it does matter. People in one study looked at real pansy flowers and silk pansies while researchers measured their heart rate variability. The people who looked at real pansy flowers showed greater relaxation responses. Gazing at realistic three-dimensional images of plants also trumps two-dimensional pictures when it comes to physiological responses. Water lilies that looked more like their in-real-life inspirations mirrored greater relaxation, measured through prefrontal cortex activity and heart rate variability, relative to looking at two-dimensional lilies. Prefrontal cortex brain activity, a measure of physiological and psychological relaxation, showed both visual stimulation and calmness in people who looked at real dracaena plants versus images of dracaena plants. Looking at pictures of nature will never have the impact of actual forest bathing in real life; they can only approximate the real thing. There is simply no substitute for authenticity.

Want to get out there in spite of your allergies? Well, we know that forest bathing likely has positive effects on your immune system. There isn't any research published yet, but maybe your immune system will improve, and so will your allergies.

WHAT IF I LIVE SOMEWHERE WITH FEW TREES?

It's true, most of the forest bathing research has been conducted in Japan, China, and Taiwan. The forests in these countries have similar properties and similar types of trees. It's reasonable to ask whether the health benefits of forest bathing would apply in other types of forests, in other types of climates. The likely answer is yes. Emerging research on exposure to blue spaces such as oceans shows health benefits similar to those from exposure to green spaces. Besides, the healing power of nature and the benefits of exposure to concordant patterns such as fractals could just as easily be accessed in the desert as in a coniferous temperate forest. It can even be found at high altitudes in the mountains.

For my husband's fortieth birthday, we planned a trip to Ecuador to celebrate together, on one of our first vacations without our kids. We spent a few days in Quito, the capital, and then traveled down the Avenue of the Volcanoes to prepare for a three-day trek up an extinct volcano named El Altar. The hike up to our first night's campsite was grueling, as we trekked through a dense bog where my foot sank several inches into the muddy ground with every step. The air was thin in the Andes mountain range and I struggled with mild altitude sickness in the form of exhaustion and a headache. Every step felt like a struggle, my feet heavy from battling the bog and my breathing slow and heavy from the lack of oxygen at the higher altitude. The last few miles felt like forever as I had to take a break to catch my breath after every single step. I could see our campsite in the distance and watched our guides set up the tents we'd be sleeping in that night. Even so, I wasn't certain I could make it.

The next day I felt a thousand times better. Having adjusted to the altitude, I felt I had enough energy to skip up the mountainside. I bounded up the trail that morning, excited to see what was beyond the ridge that had loomed above our campsite the night before. As I cleared the ridge and could see the terrain that lay beyond it, I was awestruck. Standing on the ridge revealed both the peak of the volcano and the colored lagoons fed by waterfalls, themselves fed by glaciers. The view was absolutely spectacular, which made the previous day's torturous hike worth it. We hiked along the ridge toward the glacier and the volcano's peaks, on our way to see a fifth lagoon. This last section of hiking involved scrambling through a lot of scree, small loose stones covering the slope of the mountain. I was feeling the effects of altitude again, so I opted to sit on the mountainside and wait for my group to return in a couple of hours. I sat facing the waterfall and the lagoons in the valley below me. There wasn't another human or trace of humanity around. The quietude and serenity of those few hours, without anything except a single condor soaring far off in the distance, were greater than I've ever experienced. It was truly sublime to sit, uninterrupted, with nothing except a stunning landscape to accompany me. I felt transported to another world, a world where I was merely a tourist, a tiny, imperceptible speck in a universe of giants—giant mountains and giant birds. I was far above the tree line, so technically I couldn't call it forest bathing, but the essence of the experience was the same.

HOW DO I STAY SAFE IN THE WOODS?

Overall, forest bathing is a low-risk activity with many potential benefits. It has basically no side effects, but it may need a little preparation depending on where you live, the time of year, and how long you plan on spending outside. The basics of spending time outdoors apply. If it's sunny outside, put on sunscreen. If the forecast calls for rain or snow, wear appropriate clothing. Bring enough water to stay hydrated. Snacks are always a good plan. Go forest bathing with a friend. Tell someone when and where you are going. Bring a phone in case of emergencies. Get to know the local hazards, whether they are poisonous plants or dangerous animals.

If you haven't set foot in a forest in some time, or if you've never yet visited a forest, heading out on a forest bathing session may seem a little scary. Sure, there can be hazards in the forest, but if you set out armed with a little knowledge about the natural world, the forest can feel a little bit more like a home away from home. Stay on marked trails if you aren't certain about how to identify potentially rash-inducing plants. Use caution and avoid touching plants if you aren't 100 percent clear about their safety. Wear long pants tucked into socks and closed-toed shoes to prevent irritating oils from poison ivy and poison oak from reaching your skin. Wear loose, light-colored clothing with long sleeves and pants, and apply insect repellent before forest bathing to protect yourself from getting bitten by mosquitoes. Preventive measures are especially important in avoiding transmission of mosquito-borne infections such as West Nile virus, Zika, and chikungunya. Speak to your doctor if you are considering forest bathing in areas where mosquito-borne diseases are endemic, especially if dengue, malaria, or yellow fever are present.

Tick-borne infections such as Lyme disease, Rocky Mountain spotted fever, and babesiosis are on the rise in North America, and preventing tick bites is the key to avoiding infection. The best methods of prevention are to walk in the center of trails, since ticks prefer longer grasses and leaf litter, and to follow the same recommendations for mosquitoes. If you are forest bathing in an area where ticks are known to live, do a full-body tick check when you come inside. Learn how to remove a tick safely and where to send it for testing. Ask your health care provider for details specific to your area.

Don't be afraid to turn back if needed. Even experienced outdoor enthusiasts sometimes change their plans. I was five months pregnant when we strapped our nine-month-old into a carrier on my husband's back and started off on a hike up to a series of switchbacks to a forest bathing spot with a view of the Saskatchewan Glacier in the Rocky Mountains. Weather can be unpredictable in the mountains at any time of the year and all the more so in mid-September. When we started off at the trailhead, the air was cool and the sky was mostly clear. Midway up the ridge, however, it started snowing. At first, the snow was light and fluffy. We all had on lots of warm layers, so we weren't worried about the temperature, but the snow quickly turned into near whiteout conditions. Disappointed that we had to change our plans, we turned back and slowly made our way down since we could barely see the trail. We didn't end up forest bathing by a glacier that day. Instead, we snow bathed.

More recently, I turned back on a forest bathing walk because of insects. In general, I am fearless when it comes to mosquitoes and even blackflies. They may be extremely annoying, but rarely do they get in the way of my devotion to forest bathing. That is, insects hadn't stopped me until I encountered Asian giant hornets in Taiwan. If you have never heard of them, Asian giant hornets truly are gigantic. A single hornet can grow to 1.8 inches (4.5 centimeters) long, or almost the width of my palm! And they have a monumental venomous sting to match. Although one sting isn't fatal, multiple stings can be. Asian giant hornets are responsible for about forty deaths each year in Japan alone. I'd read a lot about these deadly hornets before but had never encountered one in person until last year. I was on a short, easy forest bathing walk in the foothills of the Zhongyang or Central Mountain Range in Taiwan when I suddenly saw a massive bug fly past me. At first, I didn't believe my eyes. There are loads of large insects in Asia, and subtropical climates in general, and I am no stranger to jumbo bugs. While I paused to contemplate what kind of bug it was, another one flew close by and hovered long enough for me to clue in to exactly what it was. I confess, spotting two Asian giant hornets in a matter of seconds was enough for me to turn back and find a new forest bathing spot. I had no thought of unintentionally walking near their nest and experiencing for myself their brutal sting.

Regardless of these cautionary tales, the potential risk of spending time in nature is really quite small, especially with education around safety and environmental considerations. Be prepared, as the Scouts say, and you'll have a wonderful time. In other words, there is very little downside to nature exposure and broad potential benefits. Get outside and try forest bathing.

APPENDIX: LEARN MORE

Forest bathing resources

Association of Nature & Forest Therapy www.natureandforesttherapy.org

City Parks Alliance www.cityparksalliance.org

Forest Bathing Club www.forestbathing.club

Forest Therapy Society www.fo-society.jp/therapy/cn45/index_en.html

Healing Forest www.healingforest.org

International Society of Nature and Forest Medicine www.infom.org

LEAF—Local Enhancement & Appreciation of Forests www.yourleaf.org

National Healing Forests www.nationalhealingforests.com

National Park Foundation www.nationalparks.org

National Recreation and Park Association www.nrpa.org

Park People www.parkpeople.ca

Society of Forest Medicine www.forest-medicine.com/eindex.html

ACKNOWLEDGMENTS

To the forests of the world, thank you for being you.

To the human beings in my life, thank you for your support and encouragement as you walked with me on this path. Thank you to my mom, Maxine Kossy, for not using pesticides on our suburban lawn and for not finding the time to trim the cedar hedges. Thank you to my friend and mentor, the late Anthony Godfrey, for inviting me to cofacilitate a healing power of nature retreat early on in my career. Your love and reverence of nature was contagious and inspired me to bring nature exposure into my clinical work. To my patients, thank you for not judging me or calling me a tree hugger whenever I suggest you go hug a tree as part of your treatment plan.

Thank you to my publishing team at St. Martin's Press, especially Joel Fotinos, for knowing that I wanted to write a book on forest bathing before I did. To Gwen Hawkes, thank you for your endless patience all the times I changed my mind, and to marketing maven Jordan Hanley for ideas, motivations, and the occasional kick in the pants to be online when I just wanted to be in the woods.

Thank you to my agent extraordinaire, Suzanne Brandreth at Cooke International, for believing in my voice and recognizing the importance of a good tea selection. To Michael Tamblyn, thanks for glowing introductions that helped spark the realization that I am an author as much as I am a doctor.

Special thanks to my family for loving being outside as much as I do and walking with me off the beaten paths. To my husband, Ramesh Mantha, thank you for being my forever forest bathing partner and for magically bending space-time so that I could write, edit, and review whenever I needed. To Kirin, for singing the leaf song; and to Eli, for telling me I can do it.

INDEX

baths. *See* spas and baths
beta wave activity, 51
Beuys, Joseph, *7000 Eichen,* 67
biophilia, xii, 20
biophobia, 22
blood pressure, 29, 35–36, 70
blood sugar, regulation of, by forest
    bathing, 39
blue color. *See* green and blue of nature
body image, 48–49
bonsai and *bonkei,* 4
brain natriuretic peptide (BNP), 38
brain waves, 50–51
brain work, 43–45
breathing
    forest bathing and, 51–53
    human, mechanism of, 92–94
bristlecone pines, xxi, 72–74
bronchitis, chronic, 52
Bruce Trail, 60
Buddhism, 4, 20, 58, 96
burdock challenge game, 88
Burroughs, John, quoted, 27

cabin fever, 18
cacao tree, 90
Cameron, James, 65
camphor tree, camphor, 89
camping, 8–10, 55–56
Canada, 22, 26, 64
cancer
    low rates of, 34
    treatments for, 41
carbon dioxide, 51, 92–94
Carson, Rachel
    quoted, xi
    Silent Spring, 6
cedar wood oil, 70
ceiba (*Ceiba pentandra*), 68–69
cell service, places without, 55
chemotherapy, 41
Chicago, Illinois, 7
Chihuly, Dale, 66
Child and Nature Alliance of Canada, 7
children
    going places by themselves, 22
    nature exposure, and ADHD, 43

outside time, psychological and
    emotional development from, 53–54
playing outdoors, less in recent years,
    4–5, 21–23
Children & Nature Network, 7
children's books, 65
China, xvi
Chinese traditional medicine, xvi
chronic heart failure (CHF), 37–38
chronic obstructive pulmonary disease
    (COPD), 52–53
chronobiology, 41
cinchona trees, 89
circadian rhythms, 41, 57
cities
    feeling disconnected from nature in, 23
    planting trees in, 52
citronella, 71
citrus trees, 71
city bathing, 33
    vs. forest bathing, 48
climate change, 6
coffin tree (*Taiwania cryptomerioides*), xxi
cognitive-behavioral therapy, 49
commuting, by walking vs. by public
    transit, 110–11
coniferous forests, xxiii
conifer tree medicine, 40
conservationists, 6
coronary artery disease, 36–37
cortisol, 28–31
Cousteau, Philippe Sr, quoted, 53
creativity, 66
cypress wood oil, 70, 71
cytokines, 40–41

deciduous forests, 98
dementia, 43–45
depression, 47–48, 90
    proximity to nature and, 19
dew walking exercise, 104–6
diabetes, type 2, 39
diastolic blood pressure, 35–36
diseases, insect-borne, 119–20
dopamine, 50
Dougherty, Patrick, 67
dysbiosis, 76

ABOUT THE AUTHOR

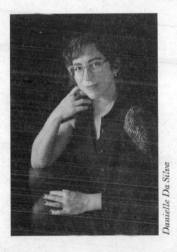

Danielle Da Silva

DR. CYNDI GILBERT, N.D., is a naturopathic doctor, author, and plant whisperer, who has been studying forest bathing and herbal medicine since she first sat under a maple tree and ate red clover flowers as a child. A faculty member at the Canadian College of Naturopathic Medicine, she taught botanical medicine and philosophy for more than ten years. She presently acts as clinical faculty at a community health center, working with underserved patients. Cyndi believes nature can inspire, rejuvenate, and connect us. She strives to bring nature into her medical practice and her everyday life.